THE NUTRITION DETECTIVE

THE NUTRITION DETECTIVE

A Woman's Guide
to Treating
Your Health Problems
Through the Foods
You Eat

NAN KATHRYN FUCHS, Ph.D.

Research Assistant—Karen Winograd
Foreword by Guy E. Abraham, M.D.

JEREMY P. TARCHER, INC.
Los Angeles
Distributed by St. Martin's Press
New York

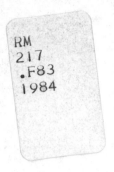
Library of Congress Cataloging in Publication Data

Fuchs, Nan Kathryn.
    The nutrition detective.

    Bibliography: p. 164
    Includes index.
    1. Diet therapy.   2. Women—Nutrition.   3. Women—
Diseases—Diet therapy.   I. Winograd, Karen.   II. Title.
RM217.F83   1984   615.8'54   85–4659
ISBN 0–87477–350–4

Jeremy P. Tarcher, Inc.

9110 Sunset Blvd.

Los Angeles, Calif. 90069

Design by Tanya Maiboroda

Manufactured in the United States of America
S 10 9 8 7 6 5 4 3 2 1

First Edition

This book is dedicated with love to the women who helped shape my life: *Shelby Victoria Robison, Anaïs Nin, Gladys Sigmund, Eileen Beaver, and Jeanette Allen, and to my nieces, Wendy and Jodi Fuchs, whose early access to this information can help shape theirs.*

CONTENTS

Foreword by Guy E. Abraham, M.D.   xi

Preface   xiii

Acknowledgments   xv

Chapter One   1
You Are Not What You Eat
    Calcium Overkill   3
    The Politics of Nutrition: Why We're Ignorant   4
    Good Health Is Balance   5
    A Woman's Life Cycle and Nutritional Needs   6
    Your Inheritance   8
    Your Lifestyle   8
    Our Allies in Health   9
    How You and This Book Can Change Your Health   9

Chapter Two   11
Becoming Aware: What You Eat Is How You Feel
    Keeping a Health Diary   11
    Interpreting Your Health Diary   18
    Cravings Versus Food Preferences   20
    Food Reactions, Symptoms, and Nutritional Causes   20
    Begin by Making Simple Changes   22

Chapter Three   24
Determining Your Biochemical Individuality
    Questionnaire Instructions   25
    Your Family's Health History   25
    Your Personal Health History   27
    Your Current Symptoms   33
    Your Reproductive System   38
    Begin Prevention the Anti-illness Way   43

Chapter Four   44
The Anti-illness Diet
    A Healthy Diet Is an Anti-illness Diet   44
    Begin with Grains and Legumes   44
    Eat a Lot of Fresh Vegetables   47
    Proteins, Our Overrated Staples   48
    Don't Forget Fresh Fruit   50
    Nuts and Seeds, the Easy-to-Carry Snack   50
    Fats and Oils, Important in Small Quantities   50
    A Practical Guide to Anti-illness Eating   51
      Breakfast, the Forgotten Meal   51
      Stop for Lunch   52

Unwind with Dinner   53
When It's Snack Time, Keep It Healthy   53
A Word About Beverages   54
And One About Cooking Utensils   54
Specific Suggestions for Meals   54
Anti-illness Recipes   57
Better Butter   57
Whole Grain Pancakes   57
Soy Milk   57
Oatmeal with Apple Juice   58
Millet with Raisins and Almonds   58
Do-It-Yourself Protein Drink   58
Vegetable Slaw   59
Hummus   59
Tabbouli   60
Pasta Primavera   60
Spicy Chinese Vegetables and Soba Noodles   61
Chicken Breasts in Wine and Tamari Sauce   61
Popcorn Supreme   61
Foods to Avoid   62
Fats   62
Sugar   63
White Flour, White Rice   64
Caffeine   64
Soft Drinks   65
Alcohol   66
Additives and Preservatives   67
Food Substitutions   68
How to Survive Eating Out   69

Chapter Five   71
Variations on a Theme
Specific Supplements Mentioned in the Diets   73
Auxiliary Treatment   77
Diets for Chronic Conditions   80
The Recovering Alcoholic's Diet   80
The Food Allergy Diet   85
The Arthritis Diet   90
The Blood Sugar Diet: Diabetes and Hypoglycemia   94
The Good Digestion Diet   100
The Fatigue Diet   103
The Headache Diet   104
The Strong Immune System Diet   108
The Healthy Skin Diet   111
Diets for the ABCs of Eating   115
The Anorexia Diet   115
The Bulimia and Compulsive-Eating Diet   117
Diets for the Reproductive System   120
The Amenorrhea Diet   120
The Candida Albicans Diet   124

The Cyst and Tumor Diet: Fibrocystic Breasts and Uterine Fibroid
  Tumors   129
The Herpes Diet   132
The Menopause Diet   135
The Menstrual Cramps Diet   137
The Osteoporosis Diet   139
The Pregnancy Diet   142
The Premenstrual Syndrome Diet   144
The Strenuous Exerciser's Diet   150
Diets for the Contemporary Woman: Minimizing the Damage   154
The Birth Control Pill Diet   154
The Caffeine User's Diet   155
The Social Drinker's Diet   157
The Smoker's Diet   158
The Stressful Living Diet   159

Afterword   162
Getting Healthy, Staying Healthy

References and Recommended Reading   164

Index   178

FOREWORD

T*he Nutrition Detective* is the outcome of five years of clinical experience and two years of extensive research of the available literature in the field of nutrition for women by an outstanding nutritionist.

It is not just another diet book. This well-conceived and detailed guide for women helps them achieve and maintain a high level of physical and mental performance. Nan Fuchs presents her approach in dealing with various situations in a very practical manner, taking into account the reader's lifestyle, dietary habits, and current health. The book is well-referenced so the reader knows which ideas and approaches originated from the author's experience and which from various sources.

The section on menopause examines the highly controversial use and abuse of calcium to prevent osteoporosis. Although an extremely high calcium diet is currently recommended by leading clinicians and nutritionists for such a condition, recent data suggest such an approach may actually be detrimental by decreasing calcium absorption and increasing soft tissue calcification. This section is particularly useful to women approaching menopause.

Ms. Fuchs should be congratulated for such perseverance and tenacity in bringing to women the new knowledge she has painstakingly gathered. Even so, nutrition is a relatively new field and a very complex one. Therefore, I would recommend the assistance of a nutritionally educated physician or other qualified health practitioner to get the most out of this book.

The Nutrition Detective is more than a woman's guide; it is a book for the rest of the family as well.

Guy E. Abraham, M.D.

PREFACE

My interest in nutrition was born out of selfishness. As a child I was criticized for being lazy because I was always tired. Allergies made me sleepy, and the allergy medication I took made me even more fatigued. Even when my allergies were under control I was prone to colds and viruses, and I was constantly bloated from poor digestion. After years of searching, good nutrition transformed me from an unmotivated, lethargic child whose nose was always running, to a vital, energetic woman. I am healthier now than I was as a teenager and stronger than I was in my twenties.

My greatest accomplishment is the happiness and fulfillment I feel, and much of this I attribute to my state of health. When I feel well, I feel strong and powerful in all areas. I am more willing to take risks and to be vulnerable, and I have more to give myself and others without feeling drained.

During my search for better health, I tried many diets that didn't work. I listened to people who claimed to have found "the answer" only to find it wasn't the answer for me. I tried a vegetarian diet and developed protein deficiencies and food allergies from eating the same items over and over. I went on a raw foods diet and suffered from gas. I tried avoiding sugar and still had no energy. Finally, I gave up in desperation and turned to stimulants—fifteen cups of coffee a day and all the sugar I wanted—and drugs. No matter what I did, my health remained the same. I was constantly bloated, gassy, slightly overweight, and lethargic, and my childhood allergies and colds accompanied me into adolescence and adulthood.

It took me years to realize I was not digesting or absorbing the nutrients from the foods I ate. It took me even longer to understand I had damaged my body with coffee and marijuana and had to repair this damage or continue to feel drained. Somewhere inside me I knew there had to be an answer. I read more books and finally began working in health-oriented businesses. During this time, I found a doctor who used nutrition as one of her primary tools. Her treatments made a tremendous difference in my health. I apprenticed myself to her for a year and a half, learning everything I could. I attended seminars on nutrition offered only to doctors and their assistants and learned there was more to nutrition than eating from the four food groups.

I was introduced to biochemists and doctors with an understanding of health who spoke of using specific foods, vitamins, and mineral supplements to enhance the body's natural ability to heal itself. I worked with other health-care practitioners whose work supported this information, and when I began working with patients, I saw how this new information transformed their lives. The information I discovered rescued me from a listless, mediocre life. Although it is not universally accepted, it is based on sound medical research and clinical observations. Its textbooks are respected journals of clinical nutrition found in all medical libraries, and its researchers are doctors and scientists with enough vision to see beyond the boundaries of the understanding of nutrition we were taught in school. In my own search, I have met some of these visionaries, attended their seminars, and taken part in some of their research.

This book is a culmination of my thirty-year search for good health that finally led me to become a nutritionist. When I first began working with patients, I realized I was more than a nutritional counselor—someone who counseled patients about an ideal dietary program. I was a detective, searching for clues to each person's health as I had for my own. The clues I found enabled me to design specific dietary programs to meet individual needs. I began calling myself a "nutrition detective."

As a nutrition detective, I help my patients pay more attention to their bodies' feedback, and I teach them how to interpret these signals. I design a program for them that will restore them to nutritional balance, allowing the natural healing process to take place. And I encourage them to become more responsible for their health. My goal is to become obsolete, to be only a resource patients can call on when they have a problem they can't solve. I am pleased to see so many of my patients relying more on themselves and becoming their own detectives, going on to solve their health problems with a new awareness.

Becoming a nutrition detective requires a specific approach, rather than a general one, along with all the data on your body you can find. This book parallels my private practice. It includes the questionnaires I have used so successfully with my patients, individual dietary programs I have developed for more than two dozen health problems common to women, and some of the most recent medical information available on the nutritional aspects of women's health care. The various programs are custom-made for you. They take into account your individual genetic makeup, as well as everything you've done to yourself in the past, from eating well and getting plenty of rest to living on fast foods and stressing your body with drugs, alcohol, sugar, and saturated fats. This book, then, is the manual you need to become your own nutrition detective.

Like me, you may have been looking for a workable solution to your health problems. Like me, you may have become dissatisfied with the general programs available until now. I am only one of thousands of women across the country who have regained their health using some of the specific methods described here. It is my hope that this book will give you the understanding and direction you need to successfully treat your health problems with nutrition, and that you can find the health and vibrancy all of us so richly deserve.

ACKNOWLEDGMENTS

I would like to thank those friends and colleagues whose support contributed so greatly to this book, in particular: Robin Raphaelian, Shelby Victoria Robison, Midge Murphy, Judy Wittenberg-Bravard, Yolanda Retter, and Stan and Mimi Reinhart. My deep appreciation for the professional assistance given so graciously by Guy E. Abraham, M.D., Uzzi Reiss, M.D., Gunnar Heuser, M.D., Loisanne Keller, O.M.D., and Dortée Farrar, Ph.D.

I have been fortunate beyond any dared dreams for the editorial wisdom and friendship of Janice Gallagher, whose clarity often exceeded mine and whose vision was always identical, and for the superb research executed by Karen Winograd.

CHAPTER ONE

YOU ARE NOT

WHAT YOU EAT

It is often necessary to make a decision on the basis of knowledge sufficient for action but insufficient to satisfy the intellect.

—IMMANUEL KANT

The area of women's health is highly controversial. We are told that premenstrual syndrome and hypoglycemia are all in our heads, that there is no way to prevent osteoporosis except by taking estrogen, and that menopausal symptoms are as inevitable as death and taxes.

We take the digestive process for granted, yet incomplete digestion often prevents the nutrients from the foods we eat from getting where they are needed. Poor digestion can be responsible for myriad health problems including compulsive eating, allergies, an inability to lose weight, bloating, fatigue, headaches, and a weak immune system.

Much of the information we have been given is outdated, and some of it is harmful. For instance, we have been told that taking additional calcium is the answer to menstrual cramps, premenstrual syndrome (PMS), and osteoporosis. Yet diets high in calcium may actually *cause* premenstrual problems, arthritis, and atherosclerosis. And taking more calcium won't prevent osteoporosis if the calcium is not able to get into the bones, a common problem among women. As we investigate the area of women's health, we must closely scrutinize each piece of information that can help us solve our own health problems. What we've been told about nutrition is not always accurate or the total picture.

Women do need calcium, but the quantitative approach to calcium represents the old nutritional approach. The "new nutrition," a qualitative approach based on sound medical research, is now available to us, although only a few orthomolecular physicians and a small number of doctors and other health-care practitioners use it in their practices. It provides us with important information that we need to become good nutrition detectives.

During the years in which I have used this new information, I have seen hundreds of women eliminate premenstrual syndrome, arthritic pains, menopausal symptoms, fatigue, and the other symptoms mentioned in this book. This new nutrition is the nutrition of the future. It is specific, sensible, possible to adapt into any lifestyle, and most important, it works. Clinical experience has shown it works not only on symptoms, but on the cause of health problems. Specific nutrition that takes into account genetic makeup brings specific results. We cannot generalize about a subject that varies so much from person to person.

To be detectives we must be thorough and look for bits of information that

1

might not appear to be important. Sometimes they are hidden, other times overlooked. My own search for good health has led me to the new nutrition. It has not been proven unconditionally, although it is well substantiated by clinical and medical research and articles that have appeared in medical journals for more than ten years. It is helping women across the country. Women who were told they needed hysterectomies have avoided surgery through better nutrition. Women who have had little energy are now leading active lives. Breast cysts and premenstrual symptoms are disappearing. Menopause has become a comfortable transition rather than a series of hot flashes and outbursts of emotion. Inexpensive and effective, the new nutrition has provided some important clues needed to solve a number of health-care problems that have plagued women for generations. It is an important aspect of your investigative work, and one of your most valuable allies in becoming a good nutrition detective.

Much of the information we have been given in the past has been incomplete. We were not told that when calcium is taken to alleviate menstrual cramps and premenstrual symptoms, the symptoms will return in following months, or that calcium malabsorption often results in osteoporosis and arthritis. Although it is true we need calcium, malabsorption often prevents it from reaching bones and cells. The issue is not how much calcium you take, but how much you are able to absorb and utilize it. *This information is not new, although it is probably new to you.* Medical research on calcium malabsorption, calcium deficiency diseases, and the overemphasized need for women to supplement their diet with added calcium has been well documented. Guy E. Abraham, M.D., research gynecologist and endocrinolgist, has surveyed medical literature for ways to treat premenstrual syndrome and has written several articles on the subject that have been published in medical journals. Fourteen years of research have led him to the startling discovery that calcium actually *causes* mood swings, anxiety, and other premenstrual symptoms. These findings are part of the new nutrition, nutritional answers to health-care problems that have not been previously solved.

Calcium malabsorption and utilization is only one problem the new nutrition can solve. Here are four primary premises to keep in mind as you begin to analyze your present state of health:

1. *You have specific vitamin and mineral requirements.*
   General nutrition is old nutrition. You are not the same as everyone else, and your needs vary greatly. Find out what foods you need to restore your body to balance and to keep it healthy.

2. *You need to be able to digest the foods you eat.*
   Without proper digestion there cannot be complete absorption or utilization. Poor digestion leaves you deficient in necessary nutrients and can either lead to health problems or prevent elimination of current problems.

3. *You do not need to take a lot of calcium.*
   You want the calcium you take to get where it is needed. Hydrochloric acid (HCl) is required for calcium utilization, and magnesium helps move calcium into bone and other cells. If you are low in any mineral, it is more likely to be magnesium than calcium. Without enough HCl and magnesium, calcium is likely to cause more problems than it can solve.

4. *You need some fats in your diet.*
   Essential fatty acids (EFAs), found in uncooked vegetable oils, are

needed by all cells and are necessary for good health. To keep slim, some women are eliminating all fats from their diet. However, a low-fat diet should include small amounts of cold-pressed vegetable oils. Premenstrual syndrome and menstrual cramps are only two indicators that you may lack EFAs.

Of these four areas, the calcium issue is undoubtedly the most startling and controversial. Doctors who use little nutrition in their practices and rely on older information learned in medical school will argue that you need more calcium. Those who read nutritionally oriented medical journals will be familiar with the approach described here. Because the calcium controversy affects most women, I have chosen to give more attention to it in this chapter. Each of the other premises is discussed in detail in chapters 3 and 4. For now, it is important to understand why you have been told to emphasize calcium in your diet, and why I, and other practitioners who are successfully using the opposite approach, disagree.

CALCIUM OVERKILL

Whatever your calcium intake, malabsorption problems may interfere with its assimilation and utilization by the body. One cause of malabsorption is the use of antacids, which decrease the HCl in the stomach needed for calcium absorption. Don't take antacids unless you *know* your body needs them. They may relieve symptoms of gastric distress that appear to be from excess HCl; however, these same symptoms may actually mean you need *more* HCl. Although you may have been told that antacids are an inexpensive way to get more calcium, this calcium is not usable because it neutralizes the HCl needed for its absorption.

Calcium absorption is definitely aided by HCl production, which is impeded not only by antacids but also by age. As we get older, our stomachs produce less HCl. This affects calcium utilization, and food digestion in general. You may not be able to digest some foods you used to eat without problems.

In addition, calcium is not efficiently absorbed when your body is deficient in magnesium, which is required for the transport of calcium into the bone and outside soft tissues, or when phosphorus intake is too high. Meat and many soft drinks are high in phosphorus and phosphoric acid; too much phosphorus pulls calcium out of your bones, causing a loss of bone density. In order for calcium to get into your bones to prevent the brittle bones of osteoporosis, it needs magnesium. If there is not enough, calcium may collect in muscles and cause cramping, it may be deposited in joints where it becomes arthritis, it can enter arteries and is called atherosclerosis, or it can cause premenstrual anxiety and moodiness, as you will see in chapter 5.

According to Dr. Abraham, in many of these conditions a diet relatively *low in calcium* and *high in magnesium* will help correct the imbalance and eliminate the problem. His research on premenstrual syndrome and osteoporosis has led him to this discovery, one I have substantiated in my own practice. Patients whose diets contain twice as much magnesium as calcium, a balance found in whole grains, for example, have eliminated health problems ostensibly solved by taking more calcium.

Magnesium, needed for calcium absorption, is largely absent in the diets of women who eat a lot of yogurt, ice cream, cottage cheese, cheese and other dairy products, and baked goods made from enriched white flour. As Dr. Abraham explains, the environment of our early ancestors was rich in magnesium and potassium, scarce in calcium and sodium. Through the decades, their bodies adapted to survive in this kind of environment. They stored calcium and sodium efficiently, and ate foods high in magnesium and potassium. Like our ancestors, we still store calcium and sodium and have to constantly replenish our supplies of magnesium and potassium. Both potassium and calcium help regulate neuro-muscular activity.

Today our diets tend to be high in calcium-rich foods like dairy products. We need to restore balance by eating more legumes, whole grains, and dark green leafy vegetables, rich in both calcium and magnesium, and less dairy. Some researchers believe magnesium may be a significant key to solving such problems as osteoporosis, menstrual cramps, muscle cramping, premenstrual syndrome, and arthritis. Chapter 4 details this Anti-illness Diet, and chapter 5 contains specific information on each of the women's health problems mentioned here.

Confusion surrounds the use of calcium, as well as other vitamins and minerals. There is confusion about which foods will best help us get and stay healthy, and which contribute to disease. There are no definitive answers to the questions that surround us, and one reason for so much confusion is the part politics plays in our health.

THE POLITICS OF NUTRITION: WHY WE'RE IGNORANT

Can dairy products cause premenstrual anxiety and mood swings? Can eating sugar cause fatigue? Is there any evidence a high-fat diet can lead to breast, ovarian or uterine cancer? Is caffeine harmful to women with breast cysts or uterine tumors? Current literature indicates strong connections between these foods and diseases. When we take a closer look at fats, sugar, refined grains (like white flour and white rice), soft drinks, caffeine, alcohol, dairy products, and food additives and preservatives, the case against eating them in large quantities is convincing. They have been linked to cancer of the breast, ovaries and uterus; heart disease; premenstrual syndrome; blood sugar imbalances; obesity; food allergies; fibroids; cysts; fatigue; headaches; digestive problems; and eating disorders. We can no longer ignore the damage they are causing simply because everyone does not agree they're harmful. The information we have been hearing for years encouraging us of their safety is based on the politics of vested interest groups and individuals.

We are caught between farmers working hard to increase their sales and profits and scientists working to solve our health problems. The billion-dollar medical research industry is geared to find cures for major illnesses, not to engage in preventive research. Much of the funding comes from pharmaceutical companies, interested in expanding their market for products rather than finding more natural ways for us to be healthy.

Political factors also influence the amount of time it takes for the results of nutritional research to reach us. For example, the dairy industry is responsible for the continued teaching of the Basic Four food groups rather than more recent information. The Basic Four program, originated in 1956 by United States Department of Agriculture (USDA) nutritionists to support agriculture, taught us to eat generous helpings of meats, grains, fruits and vegetables, and dairy products every day. In 1977, the Senate Select Committee on Nutrition and Human Needs, headed by Senator George McGovern, published a report called "Dietary Goals for the United States." This report advised us to eat less fat, cholesterol, salt, and sugar and to increase our complex carbohydrates (starches from whole grains and vegetables). This news conflicted with the Basic Four, which emphasized beef, eggs, and dairy products.

When "Dietary Goals" was released there was an outcry from farm groups. The Dairy Council and the egg and beef industries disputed the McGovern report, while others, including Dr. Siegfried Heyden, heart expert from Duke University, argued for our right to know more so we could make our own decisions based on intelligent information. Meanwhile, the USDA and the Department of Health, Education, and Welfare (HEW) held off making any comments until they thoroughly examined the McGovern report. A full two years later, each agency published separate reports which echoed "Dietary Goals." Still, nothing has changed. The Basic Four food groups are still taught in schools today.

Such a gap is not unusual. It took the Food and Drug Administration (FDA) nine years to pass a regulation making it *optional* to label fats as either saturated or unsaturated by food manufacturers so we could even know what we were eating! Although this recommendation was initiated by the FDA's top physician, it was opposed by dairies, the American Meat Institute, and other vested interest groups. Its opponents argued there was not enough proof that a high-fat diet was harmful. No such burden of proof is required in other areas of health where there are not strong special interest groups. It is not necessary to conduct sophisticated research before advising us it's smart to exercise regularly, for example. As long as these vested interest groups continue to financially support politicians we will be kept in the dark about many issues.

There is enough correlation between good nutrition and good health for you to act on now, however, and acting on it will cause fewer health problems than ignoring it. The information you have been waiting for is available. It has not been proven without a doubt, and it never will be.

The truth is, a great deal of current information is being kept from us until it is "proven" to be accurate. It has taken fifty years for the medical community to indisputably link smoking to lung cancer, and it took decades for the medical community to announce the connection between high cholesterol levels and heart disease. We don't have time to wait for this type of substantiation, nor can we afford to swallow whole the latest nutritional "cure," but going to either extreme is unnecessary.

GOOD HEALTH IS BALANCE

With the contemporary mandate to be thin, many women have turned to diets that emphasize protein, fats, or vegetables, often to the exclusion of other foods. These diets forbid certain essential nutrients and throw our bodies nutritionally off balance. Most significant, perhaps, is the fact that these diets never teach us how to eat well for our particular bodies. One popular diet based on food combining and large quantities of fruit resulted in massive sugar consumption. While fruit is certainly wholesome and contains natural sugars, women with premenstrual syndrome, hypoglycemia, and allergies found that this diet caused such problems as dizziness, fatigue, bloating, and sore breasts. A great many found that their initial weight loss reversed when they returned to eating normally.

Good health is an absence of disease and a state of balance. And balance is found in diets that contain a variety of whole foods, not a preponderance of one kind, such as the Anti-Illness Diet in chapter 4. My own clinical experience has shown me the all-or-nothing approach does not work. You don't have to be perfect to get results. Few people follow ideal diets, yet there are many healthy people who manage to eat well much of the time. Begin to make small changes knowing that every step forward is forward movement. Move at your own pace and incorporate this information gradually into your lifestyle. There is room in all the programs in this book for you to feel comfortable around food without feeling deprived or becoming a fanatic.

Although it may sound like a good idea to eat a lot of protein for weight loss, or a lot of fruit to cleanse your body, this is not always the case. Too much fruit, too much protein, or too much of anything often results in sudden weight gain once you discontinue the imbalanced diet. Good nutrition means bringing a healthy balance into your body through particular nutrients and giving your body exactly what it needs. Research indicates that since you cannot take in enough nutrients when eating junk foods or foods high in saturated fats, the ideal diet should consist primarily of whole foods. This means foods naturally grown and unprocessed (see The Anti-illness Diet, chapter 4).

Although it is easier today to buy and eat more natural foods and therefore eliminate nutritional deficiencies, it is often difficult to determine your unique nutritional needs. Your body's needs change when your reproductive system begins to function, when you are pregnant, lactating, or taking birth control pills. They change as you go through menopause and the reproductive cycle ends. Added to all of these are your individual differences, those specific to you because of inherited genetic strengths and weaknesses and your chosen lifestyle, which influences what you eat.

Perhaps you can see more clearly now that no general diet can ever hope to give you what you need and that no expert can generalize about nutrition and give you the specifics you must have to effect a major change in health. It is important to understand your individual differences and to design a specific nutritional program that will take into consideration your age, genetic individuality, any existing health problems, and the nutritional needs unique to you as a woman. Let's explore some of the ways a woman differs physiologically from a man and what these differences mean in the way you eat.

A WOMAN'S LIFE CYCLE AND NUTRITIONAL NEEDS

Whether or not you have children or intend to, your body was designed for reproduction, and the nutrients it needs to be healthy are based on this design. The stages of prepuberty, adolescence, pregnancy, menopause, and aging all require a nutritional balance specific to women. In a Harvard study, women who had 70 grams of protein a day during ages 8 to 12 produced healthier babies than those who ate less protein. (Seventy grams of protein is equal to half a pound of turkey, 1½ cups of tuna fish, or a pound of chicken breast.) This study suggests a need in growing girls for two moderate helpings of protein daily to support their bodies both as growing children and as future mothers.

With adolescence comes menstruation, a sign our reproductive system is mature. Ovulation is dependent on hormones, and to make hormones you need specific vitamins and minerals. Without these nutrients, ovulation cannot take place. Both extreme obesity and an extreme underweight condition can prevent ovulation. Because this is a time when our bodies need quantities of vitamins and minerals, adolescence is a stage when we should be eating whole, good-quality foods. Junk foods simply do not have the nutrients to give our bodies the foundation for building a healthy reproductive system.

As menstruation begins, young women have an increased need for iron. Twice as much, in fact, as men. Three-quarters of our iron is in our red blood cells, so whenever there is blood loss, as in menstruation, there is a need for more iron. Headaches, fatigue, bloating, cycles of moodiness and depression, illnesses in themselves, are now being recognized as part of premenstrual syndrome (PMS), a very real, often debilitating condition that affects thousands of women every month. PMS has specific nutritional solutions that vary according to existing physical and emotional symptoms. A description of these symptoms and their nutritional answers are found in The Premenstrual Syndrome Diet, chapter 5.

Women need even more iron when they are pregnant. The fetus's need for this mineral is so great it will take iron from the mother's body if she doesn't take in enough. During pregnancy our bodies also have increased needs for protein, calcium, zinc, copper, iodine, folic acid, and several B vitamins. While it is essential to fit these nutrients into an everyday eating scheme, it is preferable to do so under the supervision of a qualified physician or nutritionist. The Pregnancy Diet, including vitamin and mineral supplementation, is found in chapter 5.

We are also affected by the use of oral contraceptives during childbearing years. Birth control pills alter body chemistry and can change the way we metabolize carbohydrates, fats, and proteins. They can even raise blood sugar and decrease efficiency of such vitamins as B_6, B_{12}, and folic acid, resulting in some forms of PMS. By changing the hormone system, they can also cause *Candida albicans*, an insidious problem that can begin as vaginitis and spread into a complicated series of symptoms (see The Candida Diet, chapter 5). Women who take birth control pills would be wise to eat well and supplement their diet with the specific nutrients the drug depletes, as noted in The Birth Control Pill Diet, chapter 5.

At the time of menopause, which can begin from the mid-forties to mid-fifties, there is a reduction in the production of sex hormones. The level of estrogen, which helps keep our bones and tissues strong, decreases, resulting in a condition called osteoporosis. Bones become more porous and fragile, bone density decreases, and we are more prone to break bones from simple falls. This condition is three times more prevalent in women than men. Both osteoporosis and such menopausal symptoms as hot flashes, night sweats, chills, fatigue, and depression have been linked to vitamin and mineral deficiencies. Calcium, magnesium, zinc, and vitamins D, E, and B_6 should be used to support the system during menopause. Osteoporosis has been treated with estrogen therapy and increased calcium. Unfortunately, estrogen therapy can result in a higher risk of uterine cancer, and some of the latest research now shows that increased magnesium, along with exercise, may be better than large doses of calcium to help prevent bone loss as we age (see The Osteoporosis Diet, chapter 5).

Dr. Abraham, who, as a gynecologist and endocrinologist also specializes in female nutrition, believes, "A woman is fortunate. There are two times in her life when she pauses to take a good look at her diet: when she becomes pregnant, and at menopause. She becomes conscious of her diet, and she tends to eat better at these times. Men could benefit from doing this!" We can also benefit from looking more closely at other factors in our lives that contribute to specific nutritional needs.

YOUR INHERITANCE

Your diet, including any added vitamins and minerals you may need, is determined partly by your needs as a woman. It should also be determined by your genetic makeup, that is, what you inherited from your parents. We all have inherited strengths and weaknesses: good vision, strong teeth, a resistance to colds and flu, or nearsightedness, cavity-prone teeth, and a susceptibility to allergies. Your diet and added nutritional supplements can help reduce or strengthen many of your inherited weaknesses.

You need your own individualized nutritional program because your body is unique. In the 1950s, biochemist Roger J. Williams, Ph.D., conducted research that demonstrated each person's biochemical individuality. His studies proved that many people needed more nutrients than they thought, even more than the amount indicated by the RDA (Recommended Daily Allowances), which only indicates the quantity of a vitamin or mineral needed to prevent illness. It doesn't tell you how much you need to be in good health.

Becoming aware of your inherited genetic tendencies can help you take this into account in formulating an optimal health program. The questionnaires in chapter 3 have been designed to uncover specific nutritional needs based on your genetic makeup and chosen lifestyle. They take into account medication that may have upset your body's biochemical balance, as well as foods and emotional stresses.

One method for determining biochemical individuality is with the help of the Oriental medical approach. Its practitioners study pathways of energy (called acupuncture meridians) related to specific organs that are too weak or too strong in each person. Treatment using acupuncture, herbs, or massage is specific and takes into account both physical and emotional symptoms, heredity, and even the seasons of the year. In Oriental medicine, the whole person, not the disease, is treated. Although this book is primarily concerned with the way we, in the Western world, look at health and the body, it is important at times to consider the Eastern approach. For this reason, you will find references that lean heavily on Oriental medical practice and philosophy when they seem appropriate. I hope you will seriously consider these aspects of a health-care system that has worked so well for millions of people over the past five thousand years.

YOUR LIFESTYLE

In addition to the body you inherited, your dietary needs are influenced greatly by your lifestyle. A stressful job or family situation could mean you need more foods high in B vitamins, like whole grains, or extra vitamin C (see The Stressful Living Diet in chapter 5). A woman who is active in sports or exercise may need more complex carbohydrates (legumes, starchy vegetables, grains) and enough good-quality protein to support her muscle tone, as indicated in The Strenuous Exerciser's Diet in chapter 5. If you sit at a desk all day and don't exercise, you need fewer calories and would do best on a low-fat diet of high-quality foods packed with vitamins and minerals, like The Anti-illness Diet in chapter 4. The more active you are and the faster your body burns food as fuel, the more often you can eat.

How much time you have to prepare foods, what type of restaurants you frequent, and the foods your friends eat all play an important part in your food choices. Once you understand what good nutrition can do for you and how little you have to do to maintain good health, and once you achieve it, the more motivated you will be to give your body what it wants. No matter how rushed you are, you can eat well with a little advance preparation and a little guidance. Being healthy does not have to be a burden to you or the people around you, nor are you out there alone without support.

OUR ALLIES IN HEALTH

The course of nutrition today is in the hands of biochemists such as Jeffrey Bland and Roger J. Williams and medical doctors who emphasize nutrition, such as E. Cheraskin, Carl Pfeiffer, William Philpott, and Guy Abraham. These doctors are helping to develop higher standards of wellness rather than accepting the previous standards of illness. They are conducting scientific studies and drawing convincing conclusions from previous research that indicates diet is a powerful tool to lower the risk of chronic disease. They are also recommending dietary programs and supplements to eliminate deficiency diseases and for preventive purposes.

At present, Dr. Jeffrey Bland is developing a method at the Linus Pauling Institute in Palo Alto, California, by which vitamin and mineral supplements can be evaluated. His goal is to make high-quality supplements easily recognizable by giving them the Linus Pauling Seal of Quality, so we will all be able to easily distinguish the superior from the mediocre products. (See the section on vitamin and mineral supplements preceding the diets in chapter 5.)

Dr. Abraham has researched the nutritional answers to PMS for more than a dozen years and has published several articles on the subject in medical journals. His findings that a magnesium—not calcium—deficiency is responsible for many premenstrual symptoms has startled the medical community, which tends to be conservative. At the same time, the information he has uncovered has changed the lives of thousands of women who no longer suffer from PMS. Roger Williams and Drs. Cheraskin, Pfeiffer, and Philpott are only a few of the experts conducting research and writing books and scientific publications on the role the new nutrition plays in our lives. These doctors and scientists are our partners, our allies in a search for better health.

Despite this encouraging research, the majority of doctors are still slow to recognize that nutrition holds a solution for both symptoms and causes. There is now a trend to reverse this attitude. An article in *The Lancet,* a British medical journal, in December 1983, promises more emphasis on clinical nutrition for undergraduate medical students. "Of all the skills required for assessment of the individual," it states, "that of establishing food intake is the most neglected by doctors." We can look forward to doctors graduating in the twenty-first century with the proper nutritional training. Meanwhile we must take immediate action that will help us regain our health and stay healthy.

HOW YOU AND THIS BOOK
CAN CHANGE YOUR HEALTH

This book is designed to help you find the best dietary program for your body. It takes into account your family's history, your past history, your present health, and your lifestyle. The first step is to become aware. In chapter 2, you will learn how specific physical and emotional feelings can give you feedback on whether or not the foods you're eating are working for or against you.

The questionnaires in chapter 3 are to further increase your awareness and to help you plan the best diet for your particular body with its unique needs. The Anti-illness Diet presented in chapter 4 will give you the necessary guidelines to help you create a good general eating plan. This diet is often used to combat such serious illnesses as arthritis, cancer, and heart disease. You can benefit from it whether you have an illness, have a family history of health problems, or just want a good preventive program. The information you get from the questionnaires in chapter 3 will then help you modify the Anti-illness Diet for any health-care problems you may have or wish to avoid, such as alcoholism, allergies, arthritis, blood sugar problems, digestive problems, edema, fatigue, headaches, infections, eating disorders, amenorrhea, cysts, herpes, menstrual cramps, menopause, osteoporosis, premenstrual syndrome, and vaginal infections. It will also show you how to modify the diet for pregnancy and intensive exercise programs.

In addition to presenting dietary recommendations, the section on in-dividualized diets in chapter 5 contains information on nutritional supplements and adjunctive therapies. The program you design can be augmented with advice from your family doctor, nutritionist, therapist, or other health practitioner. The goal of your individualized program is to provide you with what you need to eliminate your symptoms and bring your body into greater balance.

You don't have to be sick to want greater health. You don't have to wait until you create a really big problem before you solve the little ones. The information you need to bring your body into greater balance, to good health, is not only confined to these pages. There is also a strong, loving, powerful, healthy, vital woman hiding inside you. This book will help her break through and allow her to enjoy the rest of her life.

CHAPTER TWO

BECOMING AWARE: WHAT YOU

EAT IS HOW YOU FEEL

To eat is human; to digest, divine.
— CHARLES TOWNSEND COPELAND

KEEPING A HEALTH DIARY

To begin designing your individualized nutritional program, you need to become aware of what you eat and how you feel. Since you are what you eat, digest, and absorb, how you feel is a clue to how well you eat, how completely you digest your food, and how much of these nutrients are absorbed into your cells. This will give you a better picture of your total health and will also help you analyze which foods and nutritional supplements will work best for you.

By identifying patterns, such as fatigue after eating or headaches when you skip a meal, you will have more information about which foods to avoid, which to include, and how frequently you need to eat. A detailed health diary can be a valuable tool in understanding your body and its needs if you know how to interpret it. This chapter includes instructions on keeping and interpreting your health diary.

My first step with all my patients is to have them keep a health diary for two weeks. It is often the first awareness they have of the quality and quantity of their food intake. Often a patient tells me how writing everything down helped her resist a dessert she knew wasn't good for her or made her aware of how much coffee she drank at work. You will become your body's foremost authority as you learn how to interpret its signals. These signals may be physical or emotional. Keeping a health diary is one way to differentiate between the two and become more self-sufficient.

Sometimes we dismiss physical aches, pains, and other discomforts by deciding they stem from our moods or emotions. We may have a headache from not eating and assume it was caused by an argument. Or we decide our emotional problems are physical and don't deal with our feelings. For example, when we attribute a weight-loss problem solely to the foods we eat and discount our fear of men and intimacy, we are not looking at the part our emotions play in our health.

Either approach is only part of the solution. Emotional problems can set off physical imbalances and physical problems can lead to emotional ones, but we are both physical and emotional beings at all times. And both physical and emotional aspects combine in our total health picture. It is not necessary for you to scrutinize your every feeling and try to determine the foods that caused it. Just become aware that whatever you eat may either cause or contribute to physical or emotional upsets.

A simple method is to notice how you feel from a few minutes to an hour after you eat. When you take the time to pay attention to your body, it will give you valuable information. Just as I act initially as a detective and look for patterns and relationships between emotions and food, I also teach my patients how to interpret these findings themselves.

So whether or not you *enjoy* keeping a health diary, keep one for a few weeks to allow patterns to emerge. It can teach you more about yourself than any single test or questionnaire, and you will use the awareness you gain from keeping it throughout this program. Some people go unconscious around food. Emily, a friend of mine who is overweight and can't understand why, is a good example. "I only eat two small meals a day," she insists. "I've even cut the portions in half!" I spent a day with Emily and discovered that she may eat only two *meals*, but she snacks all day long. She just doesn't count her snacks as meals. In fact, she doesn't even remember eating them most of the time! A health diary would have shown her the difference between what she was eating and what she thought she was eating.

Make enough copies of the following form (see Figure 2–1) to use for several weeks. To begin with, it is extremely important to note where you are in your menstrual cycle, since women with PMS have symptoms before their period begins that disappear as soon as it starts. If you have any PMS symptoms, it would be best to keep your health diary for three or four weeks to see how they change. Many PMS symptoms can be attributed to nutritional deficiencies or imbalances, and a combination of diet and proper nutritional supplementation can eliminate them completely.

Keep track of everything you eat, even little snacks, and note your reactions throughout the day—both physical and emotional. Make your entries when you eat or whenever you notice a reaction. It may be easier to write everything down at the end of the day, but you can't remember accurately how you felt in the middle of the morning when you're exhausted at night.

Figure 2–1 Health Diary

Number of Days Prior to Menses ___

TIME	FOOD AND WATER INTAKE	HOW I FEEL	EXERCISE
7 A.M.			
8			
9			
10			

TIME	FOOD AND WATER INTAKE	HOW I FEEL	EXERCISE
11			
Noon			
1 P.M.			
2			
3			
4			
5			
6			
7			
8			
9			
10			

There are four columns in the health diary: Time, Food and Water Intake, How I Feel, and Exercise. Fill in each of these columns independently at the appropriate time. For instance, if you have toast with butter and two eggs, orange juice, and black tea at 7:30 A.M., record them in column two. Write down everything, even if it is only a few bites. Put "water," "H$_2$O," or a check mark to indicate whenever you drink water. Do *not* write "OK," "fine," "hungry," or "full" in column three at 7:30. It doesn't give you any additional information. Look for physical or emotional feedback either before or after you eat. You may notice you feel tired or wide awake after eating; you may have indigestion; or you may have no reaction at all. If you have none, *wait until you notice a reaction before you enter anything in the third column.* Recognize whether or not you become irritable after you skip a meal.

The amount and type of exercise you get may determine in part when you eat, what you eat, and the size of your portions. To become even more aware of how much you are eating in relation to your activity, write down the amount of food and beverages in column two. Whenever you exercise, note it in column four. Write down what you do: stretch, yoga, aerobics, stationary bicycle, walk, run, jog, swim, play tennis, and so on. Indicate how long and hard you exercised. The Strenuous Exerciser's Diet in chapter 5 has more of an explanation of how to tailor the Anti-illness Diet to a heavy workout schedule. If you're not exercising, don't worry about it for now. You may be willing to when your health improves and you have more energy. In fact, at that time, it will be an important part of your total health program.

Unless you keep your diary accurately, it has little value. Figures 2–2 and 2–3 are examples of the same health diary; one kept half-heartedly, and the other kept with a whole-hearted commitment. Notice how little or how much information it can give you.

Figure 2–2 The Half-Hearted Approach

Number of Days Prior to Menses _____

TIME	FOOD AND WATER INTAKE	HOW I FEEL	EXERCISE
7 A.M.			
8	*egg / toast / juice*	*ok*	
9			
10			

TIME	FOOD AND WATER INTAKE	HOW I FEEL	EXERCISE
11			
Noon			
	sandwich & salad	fine	
1 P.M.			
2			
3			
4			
5			
6			
7	chicken /veg. /rice		
8	cookies		
9			
10			

Figure 2–3 The Whole-Hearted Approach

Number of Days Prior to Menses _____

TIME	FOOD AND WATER INTAKE	HOW I FEEL	EXERCISE
7 A.M.	1 poached egg/1 piece whole wheat toast w/ butter / 4 oz. diluted oj		
8			
	water	alert/energetic	
9			
10	water		
11			
		a little spacy irritable	
Noon	tuna salad on 2 slices w/o bread/small salad w/ oil & vinegar/1 small cookie/ herb tea	headache spacier	
1 P.M.			
		feel better / headache gone	
2	water		
3	small apple	afraid of feeling spacy again	
4			
	water		
5			
6			½ hr. aerobics class

TIME	FOOD AND WATER INTAKE	HOW I FEEL	EXERCISE
7	1 chicken breast – no skin 1 c. broccoli / ½ c. brown rice w/ Better Butter	hungry!	
8	4 lg. chocolate chip cookies	still good energy not hungry – sugar attack!	
9		very tired	
10			

The Whole-Hearted Interpretation: This is the health diary of a woman who feels best when she eats often and avoids sugar. She feels alert and energetic after a good breakfast of whole grain toast, egg, and juice, but her energy drops around 11:30 A.M., when she gets a little light-headed and irritable. These are two signs of a possible blood sugar problem. By 12:30 P.M., when she finally eats again, she has a headache and is even more light-headed. This suggests her blood sugar is low and is not providing her with the energy and fuel she needs for her brain and muscles. After eating a balanced lunch of protein (tuna fish), carbohydrate (whole grain bread), and vegetables (salad), she feels better. The sugar in the one small cookie she ate didn't seem to disturb her when it was eaten after other whole foods.

By mid-afternoon, afraid of getting some of her earlier symptoms, she ate a small piece of fruit. Apparently it worked. The fruit carried her through exercise class until dinnertime. A meal of chicken, vegetables, and brown rice kept her feeling good, but her snack of four large sugar-filled cookies a few hours later brought on exhaustion.

It would be valuable to see this person's health diary over a period of time to see if this drop in energy is an indication of a pattern. It would also be important to see it a week before her menstrual cycle to see if other patterns arise. Perhaps she craves sugar before her period and not at other times. Perhaps she has a blood sugar imbalance and needs to avoid refined foods and eat regularly on a consistent basis. I would suspect low blood sugar and suggest she explore this area more thoroughly (see questionnaires, chapter 3).

You can see by this illustration that a great deal can be learned just from looking at one day's health diary. By keeping it for several weeks, you will see patterns emerging that give you more specific, more valuable feedback about your body's relationship to food. It's now time to apply these interpretation principles to yourself.

INTERPRETING YOUR HEALTH DIARY

First, look for patterns. Some of your reactions, like fatigue or headaches, may repeat themselves. Pay close attention to the ones that appear most often, and circle or underline them with a colored pen to help you identify them. The reactions you note can have a wide variety of meanings. At first it may be difficult to interpret exactly what is going on. It can take time to become familiar with your body, its reactions, and its needs. Common patterns associated with foods include:

Fatigue after eating (sometimes or all the time)

Fatigue when skipping a meal

Headache after eating certain foods

Headache when skipping a meal

Bloating, gas, or upset stomach after eating

Depression or irritability after eating certain foods

Depression or irritability when skipping a meal

Craving particular foods (all the time or premenstrually)

Constipation

Diarrhea

Sneezing, itching, or rash after eating certain foods

Second, look for the culprit. Turn to the beginning of your diary and look for common factors. If you don't find a common denominator at first, look more closely. Your reactions may be coming either from a particular food or one of its ingredients. Sugar, salt, dairy products, wheat, or preservatives are just a few possible causes for your reactions. If you notice a reaction after eating a salad, for example, it may be coming from one of the vegetables in it, or one of the ingredients in the salad dressing. If you get symptoms after eating a sandwich, you may be sensitive to the filling or the wheat or yeast in the bread. Play detective and look for the food or ingredient that seems to be the most likely cause of the problems. Sometimes you won't know for certain, but you may have an instinctive feeling. Trust your feeling and check it out. Your body may be trying to tell you something.

Your primary problem may not be food but a lack of it. When you don't eat enough or when you skip a meal you may suffer from fatigue, headaches, irritability, nausea, dizziness, and light-headedness. Some foods don't have enough "staying power" to give you energy over a long period of time. The ones that do stick with you longest are fats (nuts, oils, butter), proteins (chicken, fish, tofu, eggs), and whole grains. They take longer to break down into sugar, the form of energy your body uses to help your brain think clearly and your muscles work well. For this reason, whole wheat-bread will give you more fuel for a longer time than a cookie made with white flour and sugar.

Third, eliminate the suspected troublemaker. Find the most obvious cause and change it. Eat a small meal instead of skipping it entirely. Try going one week without the food or ingredient you think is giving you the most trouble. Even wheat, a common ingredient in many recipes (desserts, bread, gravy, coatings) can be easily avoided with a little conscious effort (see the Food Allergy Diet, chapter 5). When you cannot eliminate a food entirely, reduce the amount you eat. Drink less coffee and soda; eat less sugar or wheat. In some cases this reduction is enough to give you relief from your symptoms. Your body may be able to tolerate a small amount of a food that produces symptoms when you eat more of it.

Fourth, look for the underlying cause and begin to change it. The bottom line for your reactions may be physical or emotional. Some common reasons for reactions to food—or not eating—are:

Too busy to eat.
Result: Skip meals and/or binge when hungry.
Solution: Make time for yourself. Eat something even if it's only a nutritious snack and not a complete meal. See the Bulimia and Compulsive-Eating Diet, chapter 5.

Too busy to prepare good food.
Result: Eat nothing, or eat junk food instead of complete meals.
Solution: Make time to nourish yourself.

Poor digestion.
Result: Feel uncomfortable and bloated, become gassy, after eating.
Solution: Chew your food well. You may also need digestive enzymes or hydrochloric acid. See the Good Digestion Diet, chapter 5, before purchasing and taking any supplements.

Craving certain foods.
Result: Give in to cravings, then feel guilty afterward.
Solution: Often comes from food allergies. See the Food Allergy Diet, chapter 5, and Cravings Versus Food Preferences in this chapter.

Eating too fast.
Result: Don't chew food well; poor digestion.
Solution: Chew more completely. See the Good Digestion Diet, chapter 5.

A history of taking antibiotics.
Result: May have caused an imbalance in your digestive tract affecting your digestion. Can cause a wide variety of physical and emotional symptoms.
Solution: May need to replenish intestinal bacteria. See the Candida Albicans Diet, chapter 5.

Don't like or know how to cook.
Result: Feel clumsy and without talent. Eat fast foods, junk foods and incomplete meals.
Solution: Ask a friend to teach you how to prepare a few dishes. Cook with someone else until you feel more confident to cook by yourself. Take a cooking class in whole-food preparation. Follow the recipes in chapter 4.

Once you begin to understand why you eat what you do and how you can change the patterns that are not working for you, you can begin putting new patterns into effect. You may see all the changes clearly before you and feel overwhelmed by them, but no one is forcing you to do them all at once—nor is this a good idea. Begin slowly, making one or two simple changes, and gradually make more changes as you feel comfortable.

CRAVINGS VERSUS FOOD PREFERENCES

Your health diary will help you distinguish between the foods you crave and the foods your body needs. One is an addiction that can lead to uncomfortable symptoms and health problems, while the other is one way your body communicates its needs to you.

Avoid the foods you crave and eat the foods you are drawn to. The distinction is subtle, but important. You will go to any lengths to get a food you crave. This is often a signal that you are addicted or sensitive to a substance and that it is throwing your system off balance. When you prefer a food, you anticipate eating it with pleasure, but are not obsessed by it. This is your body's way of telling you which nutrients it needs.

A person who can't do without coffee every day is addicted to caffeine and uses it as a stimulant. When the stimulant effect wears off, she feels tired and craves another cup. Her body knows the craving or fatigue will leave as soon as caffeine is in her system. She craves coffee to keep feeling alert, often without knowing why, without even being aware of what is going on, and she will go to any lengths to satisfy her craving. During this time she may act irrationally or become irritable, but once she has her cup of coffee she is calm, alert, and ready to continue. Cravings can occur with healthy substances, like wheat, tomatoes, chicken, nuts, cheese, and milk, as well as with unhealthy substances, like sugar, chocolate, alcohol, carbonated soft drinks, and coffee.

A person who wants a salad for lunch because it sounds appealing could probably enjoy a meal of sautéed vegetables as well, if friends and circumstances led her to a Chinese restaurant instead of a salad bar. If her body is asking for the vitamins and minerals found in vegetables, it will feel satisfied after eating them in any of a variety of forms. If it is impossible to have vegetables for lunch, she may feel less satisfied after eating and think about how to include them in her next meal.

This is a preference. Your body will tell you what it needs if you listen. It will tell you when you need more protein, vegetables, or water. It will help you differentiate between what you would "like" to have and what you absolutely can't do without. When you crave ice cream or cookies late at night and are unable to sleep because visions of chocolate invade your thoughts, you may get out of bed and find a store that's open. A craving will lead you to great lengths to satisfy it. A preference can wait until tomorrow or the next day.

The rule I use is: if you crave a particular food and nothing else will do, use all your strength to avoid it. Don't let caffeine, sugar, or a piece of bread run your life. If you are drawn to a food, if it sounds satisfying, eat it. As you keep you health diary, you'll be able to tell the difference.

FOOD REACTIONS, SYMPTOMS, AND NUTRITIONAL CAUSES.

Your need for specific nutrients and your tolerance for different foods are not the same as everyone else's. What is too much for someone else may be just right for you. This is the concept of biochemical individuality proposed in 1950 by biochemist Roger J. Williams. Your health diary will help you understand some of your needs and limitations, and the two lists that follow are broad and generalized to help you understand what may be occurring in your body.

☀ Possible Reactions to Foods ☀

Eating too much sugar or white flour could cause:
anxiety, binging, bloating, breast tenderness, depression, dizziness, edema, fatigue, headaches, increased appetite, irritability, loose stools, more energy, runny nose, sneezing, sugar craving, temporary weight gain, vaginal yeast infections

Eating too much animal fat could cause:
anger, anxiety, bloating, breast cysts, craving fats, loose stools, irritability, nausea, upset stomach

Eating too many dairy products could cause:
anxiety, bloating, body aches, breast cysts, constipation, cramps (including menstrual), craving dairy products, irritability, loose stools, mood swings, nervous tension, pain in stomach, runny nose, sleepiness, sneezing, stuffed nose, upset stomach

Food allergies could cause:
anger, anxiety, binging, bloating, constipation, craving the food you are allergic to, depression, energy, fatigue, headaches, insomnia, itching eyes, loose stools, nervousness, rashes, runny nose, sneezing, upset stomach

Too few digestive enzymes and not enough hydrochloric acid in your stomach could cause:
allergy symptoms, bloating, constipation, fatigue, frequent colds and flu, gas, headaches, loose stools, loss of appetite for proteins, nausea, upset stomach

Symptoms and Some Nutritional Causes

Achiness in joints:
citrus fruits, eggplant, bell peppers, potatoes, sugar, wheat, white flour.

Anger:
excessive fats, sugar, or alcohol; food allergy; low blood sugar.

Anxiety:
food allergy; low blood sugar; need for additional B vitamins; too many dairy products, sugar, alcohol, or white flour

Binging:
faulty digestion; food allergy

Bloating:
eating too fast; excessive fat or sugar; food allergy; not chewing well or enough; poor digestion

Breast tenderness:
caffeine; excessive sugar, salt, white flour, alcohol, or fat; need for vitamin E and essential fatty acids

21

Cramps:
   faulty digestion; high intake of dairy products (especially implicated in menstrual cramps); need for magnesium or calcium; vitamin C deficiency

Cravings:
   food allergy

Constipation:
   excessive caffeine, alcohol, or spices; food allergy; need for digestive enzymes or intestinal bacteria; need for more fluids or roughage

Depression:
   food allergy; low blood sugar; poor digestion; too much sugar or alcohol

Diarrhea:
   food allergy; food poisoning; need for intestinal bacteria; too much roughage, too much sugar or other refined foods

Eyes itching:
   food allergy

Fatigue:
   caffeine; food allergy; food preservatives like monosodium glutamate (MSG); too much sugar, alcohol, or white flour

Gas:
   food allergy; need for intestinal bacteria; poor digestion

Headaches:
   alcohol; food allergy; low blood sugar; poor digestion; sugar

Indigestion:
   eating too fast; food allergy; need for intestinal bacteria; overeating; poor digestion

Insomnia:
   caffeine; food allergy; low blood sugar; poor digestion; too much sugar or protein late at night

Irritability:
   food allergy; poor digestion; too much sugar, alcohol, or white flour

Rash or skin problems:
   food allergy; need for more water to eliminate toxins through the colon and kidneys instead of through the skin

Sneezing:
   food allergy

Stomach upset:
   food allergies; poor digestion

BEGIN BY MAKING SIMPLE CHANGES

Many of these symptoms can be caused by food allergies or food sensitivities, which may come from your body's inability to digest and absorb certain foods. Some of your discomfort, your "not feeling right," may simply be coming from a lack of digestive enzymes and insufficient hydrochloric acid. When you take care of the *cause* for these symptoms, your problems will disappear. You may want to check more carefully with your doctor, and check the Good Digestion Diet in chapter 5, before taking hydrochloric acid supplements, but you *can* begin making some changes today that could dramatically influence the way you feel.

If your list of symptoms looks alarming, begin slowly by making a few simple changes. If you can make a change safely, without any risk, do it. If you have any doubts, check them out with your doctor or health practitioner before taking any action.

Some Safe Changes Are:

1. Eat more frequently.
2. Eliminate any food that you suspect may be causing allergic responses.
3. Eat more slowly.
4. Chew your food more completely.
5. Don't drink liquids with your meal. They dilute digestive juices.
6. Eat more roughage.
7. Eliminate caffeine, alcohol, sugar, and white flour if you can.
8. Decrease your intake of caffeine, alcohol, sugar, fats, and white flour.
9. Increase your vegetables, whole grains, and water intake.
10. Eat a low-stress diet. Eat fruit alone and separate proteins from carbohydrates. This diet is easier for your body to digest than combining all kinds of foods. If you are a vegetarian, be aware that the foods you eat within a twelve-hour period are combined within your body to make complete proteins. Give your digestive system a rest.

After you make the changes you can, keep your health diary for another two weeks. Sometimes you will see a dramatic reduction in symptoms within a day or two. Other times it may take a few weeks or even a few months before your symptoms are alleviated or gone. Notice how aware you are now compared with when you first began. As you use your diary more, this awareness will continue to grow. Even if you haven't yet found all the answers to your health problems, you've made an important start with the help of your diary. You know your body has its own particular needs, and you know how to begin fulfilling them. You know there is a relationship between what you eat and how you feel.

The health diary is one of several tools you can use to help determine your specific needs. The questionnaires in chapter 3 will carry your understanding of your biochemical individuality—what makes your needs different from someone else's—even further. The answers to these questionnaires will help you choose the specific diets in chapters 4 and 5 that will bring you to a higher state of health.

CHAPTER THREE

DETERMINING YOUR

BIOCHEMICAL INDIVIDUALITY

*Strange! all this difference should be
'Twixt Tweedledum and Tweedledee.*
—JOHN BYROM

This chapter contains four questionnaires, including a brief family health history, your personal health history, your current symptoms, and a section relating to your reproductive system, to help you learn more about your body. The interpretation section following each questionnaire indicates the appropriate modifications in diet for your particular problem. These modifications will combine to provide the most nutritious diet for *your* body at this time of your life.

As you complete the questionnaires, a profile will emerge that is uniquely yours, indicating how your health has been affected by past accidents, illnesses, the stresses of living, and your family's eating habits; what your current state of health is; and what may be in store for you. You will get the most accurate assessment of your health possible if you fill out all the questionnaires as completely as you can.

Your Family's Health History provides a genetic overview of your family, indicating weaknesses you may have inherited. When several relatives have had the same illness, it may indicate a genetic predisposition for that illness in other family members. Often, a history of alcoholism, diabetes, hypoglycemia, premenstrual syndrome, osteoporosis, heart disease, or cancer is accompanied by poor family eating habits. When a family tends to eat a high-fat diet, breast cancer and coronary heart disease are not unusual. When they eat a lot of refined foods, blood sugar problems and premenstrual syndrome is understandable. While particular illnesses are not necessarily inherited, a genetic weakness for these illnesses may be, and the foods you have been brought up eating and have learned to enjoy may push you over a precarious edge into symptoms and health problems.

This questionnaire also helps you look closely at the health patterns of the relatives you most resemble, physically and emotionally. Since your health could imitate theirs, you may want to alter your patterns for the better.

Please note that this questionnaire is a screening device to make you more aware of your family's health and your tendencies to develop some of the health problems that seem to recur in your family. It is not intended to alarm you. Rather, when you are more informed, you can adapt the Anti-illness Diet accordingly. It is simple to create a nutritional program to avoid particular health problems when you are clear about your goals.

Your Personal Health History shows you how you have treated your body throughout your life. It surveys illnesses that may have weakened it and looks at the medications you have taken, as well as such habits as smoking and drinking alcohol or caffeine. And it gives you the opportunity to take a look at the amount of sugar, fat, and salt you eat. It also reveals the long-term effects of such events as injuries, surgeries, and exercise programs.

Your Current Symptoms goes beyond your primary complaints to focus on all the little "unimportant" symptoms that are your body's way of communicating to you what's going on. This questionnaire is helpful in identifying both current and future health conditions.

Your Reproductive System, the final questionnaire, is presented in greater detail because many of your past, present, and future health problems revolve around your body's ability to bear children. The hormonal changes associated with menstruation and menopause result in specific nutritional needs unique to women. Stress, vaginal infections, amenorrhea, a constant need to replenish the iron lost each month through menstruation, and your body's ability to absorb calcium to prevent menstrual cramps, premenstrual syndrome, osteoporosis— these are all part of a woman's health-care picture.

QUESTIONNAIRE INSTRUCTIONS

Begin by making photocopies of each questionnaire, then answer each question as completely as you can. If you don't have enough information and a phone call will provide you with additional data, take the time to make that call. If it would require writing someone in your family, you may want to wait before taking the time to write. Some questions will be more pertinent for you than others. When you can't answer a question, leave it blank.

When you have completed the questionnaires, review them, looking for recurrent health problems. These will be areas to look at more carefully in light of preventive health care. You may have a primary complaint, or maybe several symptoms and clues fit together to give you a clearer picture of what to do next. For many women, the first step is to begin with the Anti-illness Diet in chapter 4. If you like, you can then alter this diet to work with specific health problems or for preventive purposes according to the modifications found in chapter 5.

YOUR FAMILY'S HEALTH HISTORY

1. How many of your blood relatives (parents, grandparents, aunts, uncles, cousins, brothers, sisters) have had the following:

Alcoholism _____	Hypertension _____
Arthritis _____	Hypoglycemia _____
Cancer _____	Kidney Problems _____
Diabetes _____	Liver Problems _____
Gall Bladder Problems _____	Mononucleosis _____
Heart Disease _____	Osteoporosis _____
Hepatitis _____	Premenstrual, Menstrual, or Menopausal Problems _____

2. List your father's major health problems: _____

_____

3. List your mother's major health problems: _____

_____

At the time your mother conceived and was pregnant with you, did she: use drugs or other medications, drink alcohol, eat a lot of sugar, drink a lot of coffee or black tea, or have a generally poor diet? _____

_____

4. List your grandmothers' and grandfathers' major health problems (include cause of death if applicable): _____

_____

5. List your aunts' and uncles' major health problems: _____

_____

6. How long do the women in your family tend to live? _____

7. Who in your family do you most resemble physically? _____
   Describe his/her condition of health: _____

_____

8. Who in your family do you most resemble emotionally? _____
   Describe his/her condition of health: _____

_____

Interpreting Your Family's Health History:

Question 1: If two or more blood relatives have had the same health problem, a hereditary weakness may be indicated. This is a signal for you to pay attention to a dietary program that is least likely to allow this weakness to occur in you. A word of explanation about mononucleosis is necessary. Mononucleosis often results in a low immune system. If some relatives have had severe cases of mononucleosis, find out whether or not they have had any illnesses that are associated with low immunity, such as colds, flu, allergies, and even cancer and arthritis.

Questions 2 and 3: Your parents' health can influence yours. If one or both are overweight, have high blood pressure, or other problems, look at these areas in your own life, especially if your living and eating habits are similar. Your mother's health at the time of your conception and during pregnancy could also influence yours. Many babies are born with drug dependencies, a weakness in their blood sugar balance, and liver and other organ weaknesses that come from their parents. Hyperactivity, cervical cancer, and slow mental development have been linked to the ingestion of drugs such as DES, caffeine, cigarettes, and alcohol during pregnancy.

Questions 4 through 6: A close look at your relatives' health and longevity can give you clues about possible inherited strengths and weaknesses. If all the women in your family live to a ripe old age, it *could* mean you're getting ready to follow in their footsteps. If they have arthritis, osteoporosis, or diabetes, you may want to set up a preventive program for yourself.

Questions 7 and 8: You are more than your parents' child—you are part of two families with their separate health histories and patterns. When you stop to analyze your health profile, you may find it is similar to that of the one or two relatives you tend to resemble most, both physically and emotionally. Be aware that genetic tendencies like diabetes can jump a generation and also that this tendency does not guarantee you will or will not contract the same health problems as your relatives. These are simply things to consider and be aware of.

YOUR PERSONAL HEALTH HISTORY

1. Have you had measles? _____ mumps? _____ chicken pox? _____

2. Have you had any unusual childhood diseases (diptheria, scarlet fever, and so on)?

   _____

3. Have you had mononucleosis? _____ hepatitis? _____ other major illnesses (list them)? _____

4. List all surgeries (including tonsillectomy, appendectomy, cesareans, abortions and so on):

   _____

   _____

   _____

   _____

5. List any major injuries, including heavy blows to the head (falls, auto accidents, and so on): _____

   _____

   _____

6. List all present medication (prescription or over-the-counter): _____

   _____

   _____

7. List any recreational drugs you now use (marijuana, cocaine, and so on):

   _____

   How often do you use them? _____
   In what amount? _____
   List any you have used for six months or more on a regular basis (four times a week or more): _____
   How much did or do you use per day/week/month? _____

8. List all vitamins and minerals you are now taking and why:

Supplement	Dosage	Reason
_____	_____	_____
_____	_____	_____
_____	_____	_____
_____	_____	_____
_____	_____	_____
_____	_____	_____
_____	_____	_____
_____	_____	_____

Do you notice any improvement in the way you feel since you began taking them? _____
Have you noticed any undigested supplements in your stool? _____

9. List any known allergies (to pollens, dust, food, petrochemicals, medications, and so on): _____

_____

10. Do you smoke cigarettes? _____ If so, how many per day? _____
Did you ever smoke heavily in the past? _____ For how many years? _____ Do you live or work with someone who smokes frequently? _____

11. Do you drink alcohol? _____ If so, how often?_____
What do you drink (beer, wine, hard liquor)? _____
How many drinks do you have daily, weekly, or monthly? _____
Did you ever drink heavily in the past? _____ For how many years? _____

12. Do you drink caffeinated drinks (coffee, black tea, colas, hot chocolate)? _____ How many cups/glasses a day, combined? _____
Did you ever drink caffeinated drinks heavily in the past?_____

13. Do you drink decaffeinated coffee? _____ How many cups per day? _____

14. Do you add salt to your food? _____ Do you eat salty foods often? _____

15. Do you add sugar to your food? _____ Do you eat sweet foods often? _____

16. Do you eat more than one serving of dairy products a day (milk, cheese, cottage cheese, yogurt, ice cream, ice milk)? _____

17. Do you prefer foods that are salty, sweet, or fatty? _____

18. Do you get tired after eating? _____ If so, how often? _____

19. Do you drink water daily? _____ How much? _____ When? _____

_____

20. Do you exercise regularly? _____ If so, how often? _____
What kind (swim, walk, jog, aerobics, bodybuilding, and so on)? _____

_____

If not, why not (too tired, busy, or lazy; back or other injuries; not
motivated; and so on)? _____
Would you exercise if you had more energy and felt better? _____
What kinds of exercise would you be willing to do? _____

_____

Interpreting Your Personal Health History:

Questions 1 through 3:   Childhood diseases and serious illnesses can lower
your immune system, leaving your body with hidden weaknesses in areas you
never suspected. These weaknesses can lead not only to frequent colds and flus,
but also to allergies and digestive problems. Large or frequent doses of antibiotics
can also affect your health. They can disrupt the bacterial balance in the colon and
vagina, and cause diarrhea, vaginal infections, and more. Further information on
some of the consequences of antibiotics is found in the Your Reproductive System
questionnaire in this chapter.

Measles, accompanied by a high fever, could affect your heart or cause skin
problems later in life. Chicken pox can lead to such viruses as herpes zoster (cold
sores) or shingles. Hepatitis, an inflammation of the liver, often results in long-
lasting sensitivities to alcohol and drugs and a liver that will benefit from a
supportive diet free of chemical additives and other toxins (see the Healthy Skin
Diet, chapter 5).

Question 4:   As with childhood and other illnesses, look to the cause for and
the effect of your surgery. If it was not due to an accident, look for the most
probable cause or the area of primary concern. For example, a hysterectomy
could have been performed due to enlarged uterine fibroid tumors. If so, note the
similarities between breast cysts and uterine tumors (chapter 5) to see which
dietary factors might have contributed to the fibroids that could also affect the
formation and growth of breast cysts.

Look closely for the cause for your surgery. It solved a problem temporarily
by removing it from your body, but this does not prevent it or a related problem
from recurring. The surgery may have deprived your body of important functions.
The removal of tonsils or appendix could result in lowered resistance to infection
because the body is deprived of part of its filtering system. Complete hysterectomies result in hormonal changes. Other surgeries of the reproductive system can
be a sign of chronic infections or poor nutrition that point to a need for improved
nourishment to prevent further problems. Use this question to look for indications of a pattern that may be clearly present or starting to emerge.

Question 5:   Past injuries can be responsible for present or future health
problems. Any injury to the spinal column can affect the health and integrity of
nerves, which feed all your organs and glands. They can cause indigestion,
reproductive-system weaknesses, and myriad other symptoms. Some health problems may stem from old injuries or accidents. In these cases, even the best
nutritional program will not help until the underlying cause is corrected. If your

problems do not respond to dietary changes, consult an osteopath or chiropractor who can look for, and treat, structural problems.

Questions 6 and 7: Drugs are chemicals and interfere with your body's natural functions. Many prescription and over-the-counter drugs are specifically designed to stop, slow down, or speed up body functions. You may have been asked to use drugs temporarily to help your body regain its health and balance. Look at the underlying reason you are taking these drugs to see if there is a nutritional alternative. Check with your doctor to see if it is safe to try.

Taking some drugs can initiate problems. Antacids, for example, can result in a low iron count due to a malabsorption of iron, which requires hydrochloric acid in the stomach for its absorption. If you are taking antacids for poor digestion, read the Good Digestion Diet in chapter 5. Birth control pills have been implicated in headaches, vaginal infections, and nutritional deficiencies. If they are your choice of contraception, supplement your diet with the vitamins and minerals listed in the Birth Control Pill Diet in chapter 5. Tetracycline and other antibiotics can slow down protein synthesis and destroy helpful bacteria in the colon, resulting in diarrhea and other intestinal problems. This bacterial balance can be restored by taking acidophilus capsules or by eating yogurt. Antibiotics can also lead to vaginal infections like *Candida albicans,* or monilia. Because *Candida* can cause myriad women's health problems, refer to the Your Reproductive System Questionnaire in this chapter and the Candida Albicans Diet in chapter 5.

It is impossible here to note all possible effects of prescription drugs you have taken in any significant amount over the years, but if you are interested in knowing more, look through a recent volume of the *Physician's Desk Reference* (PDR), which lists all known harmful effects.

Recreational drugs, including marijuana and cocaine, also affect your health. According to the textbook *The Pharmacological Basis of Therapeutics*, the tar from marijuana has been found to be more carcinogenic than cigarette tobacco. Even relatively small amounts could add up to problems over time. In addition, my clinical observations over the past eight years indicate people who smoke marijuana consistently for six months or longer exhibit some form of blood sugar imbalance, including premenstrual sugar craving and binging, headaches, and fatigue (see the Blood Sugar Diet, chapter 5).

Although cocaine does not appear to affect blood sugar, it overstimulates the brain and may cause brain cell destruction by toxic overdose. In addition, it causes inflammation in nasal tissues and affects the sinuses. It is difficult to determine how much cocaine is harmful, partly due to individual tolerance levels. However, overwhelming evidence points to side effects in long-term use of amphetamines, barbiturates, and other self-administered drugs. My recommendation to all health-conscious people is to stop using them.

Question 8: Vitamins, minerals, and other nutritional supplements could be helping your health or contributing to its decline. If your supplements are being eliminated in your stool, they are not doing you any good at all. Like food, they must be broken down and absorbed first. If you *think* your supplements are causing any problems such as nausea, headaches, or fatigue, stop taking them for a few days to see if the reactions leave. The complex subject of nutritional supplements is discussed in detail in chapter 5. You will want to read that section thoroughly before buying or replacing any supplements to understand the importance of buying high-quality supplements, which are often absorbed more easily than bargain brands.

Question 9: Allergies or sensitivities can be inherited or acquired by repeated exposure to a food or chemical. In many cases they are caused by digestive problems. If you can't digest your food, your body treats the undigested particles as foreign substances and you have an allergic reaction. Refer to the diets on allergies, the immune system, and digestion in chapter 5 to see which applies best to you.

Question 10: Smoking can cause or contribute to allergies, affect your lungs, and add toxic metals like arsenic, cadmium, and nickel to your liver. Some studies link smoking to lower estrogen levels and osteoporosis. Nicotine is present in breast milk and can affect nursing children. In addition, smoking contributes to heart disease, problems handling blood sugar, and is strongly implicated in cancer of the cervix. It also weakens your immune system. If you are not a smoker but live or work with someone who is, you are a passive smoker. The fumes you inhale may be as toxic as though you smoked. Research shows that antioxidants, particular vitamins and minerals, help both the smoker and the person who inhales secondhand smoke. If you are either an active or passive smoker, see the Smoker's Diet, chapter 5, for nutritional supplement recommendations.

Question 11: Alcohol affects blood sugar levels, the absorption of vitamins and minerals, and is believed to affect the fetus in mothers who drink ten drinks or more a week. As a sugar, it contributes to some forms of premenstrual syndrome and encourages the growth of infections, including *Candida albicans* and herpes. It aggravates arthritis, contains yeast and other substances that can cause allergic reactions, and contributes to edema, headaches, and a low immune system. Low levels of alcohol may not cause any problems unless your liver has been weakened by hepatitis. If you drink regularly, you may want to evaluate the following programs: The Headache Diet, the Strong Immune System Diet, the Recovering Alcoholic's Diet, the Social Drinker's Diet, the Food Allergy Diet, the Premenstrual Syndrome Diet, the Candida Albicans Diet, and the Blood Sugar Diet, all in chapter 5.

Questions 12 and 13: Caffeine is strongly linked to bladder cancer, pancreatic cancer, fibrocystic breasts, and uterine fibroids. If you have cysts of any kind, caffeine should be eliminated from your diet. It can also irritate ulcers, contribute to anxiety and fatigue, cause headaches, heartburn, hypertension, blood sugar problems, and birth defects. It affects fatty acids in the blood and can contribute to high cholesterol. Decaffeinated coffee contains only small amounts of caffeine but may still cause heartburn, which is often caused by increased gastric acids and a relaxing of pressure in the esophagus. Both types of coffee can contribute to poor digestion. Decaffeinated brands may also contain chemical residues toxic to the liver. The caffeine in soft drinks, black tea, and certain herb teas like maté and guarana, is as harmful as caffeine in coffee. Guarana is an herb used in some appetite suppressant and energizing formulas. Chocolate contains smaller amounts of caffeine, which can still be significant if you eat large quantities. Although caffeine contributes to a wide variety of complaints, the most pertinent diets to review include the Blood Sugar Diet, the Cyst and Tumor Diet, the Fatigue Diet, and the Caffeine-user's Diet, chapter 5.

Questions 14 through 17: Overconsumption of salt, sugar, and dairy products can all contribute to health problems. Each person has a unique tolerence level for these substances. Refer to the Anti-illness Diet in chapter 4 for ways to use them without abusing them.

Salt can contribute to hypertension and premenstrual symptoms such as tender breasts, bloating, weight gain, and edema. A craving for salt could indicate tired adrenal glands, meaning you're under too much stress. When the stress is reduced (through diet, relaxation techniques, exercise, solving the problems that are causing it, and so on) the salt craving diminishes. See the Premenstrual Syndrome Diet in chapter 5. The Anti-illness Diet in chapter 4 is also an anti-stress diet.

Elevated sugar levels are often found in recovered alcoholics. Since alcohol is absorbed directly into the bloodstream, people who stop drinking may continue to crave sugar in other forms like candy, cakes, doughnuts, cookies, added to coffee, and so on. Sugar disrupts the blood sugar balance and can lead to hypoglycemia or diabetes. It is a major source of edema, causing the kidneys to retain fluid. It also contributes to a number of premenstrual symptoms. Sugar feeds infections, especially yeast infections, and can cause headaches and digestive problems like gas and diarrhea. Many people are addicted to sugar, and food addictions often signal allergies. Most important, eating large amounts of sugar can take the place of eating more nutritious foods and indirectly lead to severe nutritional deficiencies. See the Recovering Alcoholic's Diet, the Blood Sugar Diet, the Fatigue Diet, the Strong Immune System Diet, the Bulimia and Compulsive-Eating Diet, the Premenstrual Syndrome Diet, the Candida Albicans Diet, and the Social Drinkers's Diet in chapter 5.

Dairy products are a double-edged sword. They are high in animal fats, calcium, and lactose. Since calcium is so difficult for many women to utilize, an excess of dairy products can contribute to arthritis, atherosclerosis, premenstrual anxiety and mood swings, menstrual and other types of cramps, and osteoporosis. Its high fat content makes it an undesirable food for women with breast cysts or uterine fibroids and anyone with high cholesterol. Dairy allergies are among the most common, and dairy products can contribute to digestive problems, headaches, and compulsive eating. Lactose increases urinary excretions of magnesium and increases your body's demand for magnesium. See the Food Allergy Diet, the Cyst and Tumor Diet, the Menstrual Cramps Diet, and the Premenstrual Syndrome Diet, chapter 5.

Question 18: Fatigue from a few minutes to several hours after eating is a sign of digestive problems or food allergies. Pay attention to how you feel after a meal or snack. You may get tired after every meal or only occasionally when you eat certain foods. If you have this symptom, see the Food Allergy Diet and the Good Digestion Diet in chapter 5.

Question 19: Drinking half a glass of plain, purified water every hour will solve more problems and eliminate more symptoms than you can believe. Water is absorbed into your body through the colon and helps flush toxins and other wastes out of the body through the kidneys. Low back pain is often a sign your kidneys need more water. Constipation can be a signal that your body needs more water and has taken some of what it needed from your colon, leaving you with hard, dry stools. Skin problems may be caused by toxins leaving your body the only way they know how when they're not being eliminated through the kidneys and colon. Don't drink water or other liquids half an hour before or after meals. It dilutes the hydrochloric acid in your stomach and can contribute to digestive problems. Instead, chew your food well to provide enough moisture and limit your liquids with meals. For more information on skin problems, refer to the Healthy Skin Diet in chapter 5.

Question 20: Twenty minutes of aerobic exercise three or four times a week strengthens your heart, provides you with additional energy, reduces your appetite, and changes your metabolism so you burn food more quickly. Aerobic exercise is some form of exercise where your muscles are continuously working for at least twelve minutes. Brisk walking, jogging, running, stationary bicycling, bicycling, rowing, trampoline, jumping rope or jumping in place, and cross-country skiing are aerobic. Most other exercises are not, no matter how vigorous they seem. Exercise is nutrition for your muscles and cardiovascular system. It should be combined with your Anti-illness Diet to form a complete anti-illness program.

A brisk walk outdoors daily has been found to help eliminate premenstrual anxiety and moodiness. Exercise is especially important for all women concerned with getting osteoporosis. Weight-bearing exercises like walking, jogging, and aerobics classes help keep bones dense. If you are not exercising now, it is important to begin as soon as you start feeling well enough. It keeps body fat, including cellulite, low, tones muscles, and keeps your body younger and more flexible. See the Osteoporosis Diet, the Premenstrual Syndrome Diet, and the Strenuous Exerciser's Diet, chapter 5.

YOUR CURRENT SYMPTOMS

Check all symptoms you've experienced two or more times a week over the past three months, or that are part of an ongoing problem.

1. **Your Digestive System (breakdown of foods):**
   Have an excessive appetite _____
   Have gas _____
   Have indigestion, fullness or bloating after eating _____
   Don't have much appetite for meat or other protein _____
   Get tired after eating (always or occasionally) _____
   Have a history of anemia _____
   Stool has a foul odor _____

2. **Your Liver and Gall Bladder (fat metabolism):**
   Have light-colored stools _____
   Have difficulty digesting fatty foods _____
   Have, or have had, hemorrhoids or varicose veins _____
   Have had jaundice or hepatitis _____
   Have eye problems (other than near- or farsightedness) _____
   Have pain or sensitivity under the right ribs _____

3. **Your Intestines (absorption and elimination):**
   Have constipation _____
   Have used antibiotics recently, or in large amounts in past _____
   Have long, thin stools _____
   Notice undigested food particles in stool _____
   Have more than three bowel movements a day _____
   Have colitis or diverticulitis _____
   Have skin problems _____

4. Your Blood Sugar (energy):
   Become irritable before meals _____
   Get shaky when hungry _____
   Have low energy in the afternoon, or are generally fatigued _____
   Wake up at night and find it difficult to go back to sleep _____
   Crave sweets, starches, or alcohol _____
   Get depressed _____
   Skip meals _____

5. Your Adrenal Glands (body's ability to handle stress):
   Eyes sensitive to light _____
   Become dizzy when you stand up suddenly _____
   Have frequent pain or weakness in your knees or low back after exercising _____
   Have a history of allergies and/or hay fever _____
   Crave salty foods _____
   Have menopausal symptoms _____
   Are a perfectionist or workaholic _____

6. Miscellaneous Symptoms:
   Get headaches _____
   Get frequent colds and/or flu _____
   Feel run-down _____
   Feel like you're under constant stress _____
   Have swelling or pain in joints or neck _____
   Feet and fingers feel swollen or bloated _____
   Feel fat even when others tell you you are thin _____
   Eat very little, always on a diet _____
   Binge and vomit _____
   Eat constantly, even when not hungry _____

Interpreting Your Current Symptoms:

Your Digestive System: This section gives many clues about your body's ability to use the foods you eat. Your stomach may not produce enough hydrochloric acid to help break down food, or your pancreas may not make enough enzymes to continue the digestive process started in the stomach. Although the food may never get small enough to be absorbed into your cells, when you eat your body *thinks* it has received particular nutrients because, through chewing, your brain has been told by your taste buds that digestion is about to take place. When it finds out it has been fooled, it demands more food in an attempt to get the vitamins, minerals, and other building blocks it needs. Compulsive overeating or craving particular foods may be the result.

Question 1: If you're not eating out of habit or frustration, an excessive appetite could mean you're not digesting your food completely. A number of other symptoms could indicate you don't have enough hydrochloric acid in your stomach: gas, indigestion, bloating after eating, little appetite for meat and other proteins, a history of anemia, and calcium absorption problems. To be absorbed, calcium requires stomach acidity in the form of HCl. For further discussion on calcium malabsorption, see the Osteoporosis Diet, chapter 5. Indigestion, bloating, and gas can also mean insufficient enzyme production by the pancreas, and foul-smelling stool indicates incomplete digestion. For advice on how to create a program to solve your digestive problems, see the Good Digestion Diet, chapter 5

Your Liver and Gall Bladder: The liver is like a large chemical factory. It stores and releases sugar, sends toxic wastes down to the kidneys and colon to be eliminated, stores whatever toxins it doesn't know how to eliminate, manufactures some essential hormones like estrogen, and produces bile, a liquid that helps dissolve fats, and sends it to your gall bladder for storage. In addition, it performs hundreds of other chemical functions. The liver is damaged by alcohol, too many fats, and a wide variety of toxic materials. Some of these come from additives or preservatives in the foods we eat, and some from the environment—like exhaust fumes, tobacco smoke, insecticides, pesticides, gasoline and paint fumes, and even hair spray.

The liver is a marvelous workhorse. It can function even when it is congested with toxins and congealed with fat. But this can cause secondary symptoms like fatigue, hemorrhoids, blood sugar imbalances, and premenstrual problems. Because the liver continues to function even when it is overworked, a blood test is often the only way to get the true picture of how it's doing. At other times, the liver gives us clues. If you suspect your liver and gall bladder need a gentle cleansing, refer to the Healthy Skin Diet, chapter 5, for a detoxification diet that will benefit both your liver and skin.

Question 2: Light-colored stools indicate a problem digesting fatty foods or an excess of fats in the diet. In either case, eating less fat and possibly taking digestive enzymes could be helpful. More specific information is located in chapter 5 in the Good Digestion Diet and the Healthy Skin Diet.

Hemorrhoids are varicose veins in the colon caused by a congested liver, which puts pressure on the portal vein, a vein that goes from the colon to the liver. The same kind of pressure in other veins produces varicose veins. Both may stem from liver congestion. Jaundice and hepatitis can affect the liver's health for many years. If you have had either illness and continue to eat foods high in fat or drink alcohol, you may be causing additional damage.

For centuries, Oriental medicine has linked the eyes with the liver. The acupuncture meridian (a pathway of energy) for the liver ends at the eyes. An imbalance along that pathway may affect either the eyes or the liver. If you have noticed any unusual impaired vision that does not come from being either near- or farsighted, first have your eyes checked by an optometrist or ophthamologist to rule out pathological problems, then clean up your liver. Many of my patients report fewer eye problems after going on a detoxification program (see the Healthy Skin Diet, chapter 5).

A pain or sensitivity under the right ribs is an indication the liver is swollen from disease or improper diet. Since it repairs itself rapidly and can regenerate cells, a good diet like the Anti-illness Diet in chapter 4, regular exercise, and plenty of rest can turn a weak liver into a strong one.

Your Intestines: Even with enough fiber in your diet, you can be constipated if your water intake is low. If you don't drink enough water, your body will obtain it from the large intestines (colon), where water is absorbed into your body, and leave you with dry, hard stools. You need both enough fiber and water for good elimination.

Question 3: Long, thin stools, undigested food particles, or many bowel movements can mean poor digestion or poor absorption through the walls of the small intestines. Colitis (inflammation of the colon) or diverticulitis (inflammation of a sac in the colon) may indicate there is not enough roughage to push wastes through, too many refined foods like sugar and white flour, or improper digestion.

When there is poor elimination of wastes through the kidneys and bowels, toxins have no way to leave the body except through the skin, your largest organ of elimination. While there may be many causes for skin problems, they may simply be your body's way of telling you to drink more water or clean up your diet. If the Anti-illness Diet in chapter 4 does not make a significant change in the condition of your skin, you may want to modify that diet according to the Healthy Skin Diet in chapter 5.

Your Blood Sugar: Much of your energy is regulated by the balance of sugar in your blood, which feeds your brain and muscles. Insulin, a protein produced in the pancreas, helps your body use, store, and eliminate excess sugar. It helps move sugar into and out of the liver, where extra glucose is stored, and sends it where it's needed. Eating excessive amounts of carbohydrate can throw off the pancreas's insulin-regulating mechanism and leave you with too much or too little sugar, causing either hypoglycemia or hyperglygemia (diabetes). Because the Anti-illness Diet does not contain refined foods, it is a good place to begin if you suspect any kind of blood sugar imbalance. For more specific information, refer to the Blood Sugar Diet, chapter 5.

Question 4: Some signs of blood sugar imbalances can be a feeling of irritability or shakiness when you're hungry, feeling tired around mid-afternoon when your sugar supply has run out, or a constant feeling of fatigue. This is when you may crave sweets, starches (which turn to sugar), or alcohol the most. Eating complex carbohydrates (whole grains in any form) will often alleviate these cravings, since they turn into sugar more slowly. If your cravings are frequent, you may need to eat more protein. See the Blood Sugar Diet, chapter 5.

If you wake up at night, your blood sugar may be low. Low blood sugar levels can cause extreme hunger in the middle of the night or in the early morning hours. In such instances, eating a little protein or taking a complete amino acid formula (predigested protein) in the evening can enable you to sleep comfortably through the night. See the Blood Sugar Diet, chapter 5.

Depression can come from many causes, including alcoholism and blood sugar imbalances. I have seen numerous cases where depression vanished as soon as a person's blood sugar became more even. If you skip meals you may run out of sugar (energy) and contribute to blood sugar irregularities. One way to keep your blood sugar level is to eat small meals throughout the day and to follow The Blood Sugar Diet in chapter 5.

Your Adrenal Glands: There are all kinds of stresses in our lives, and our adrenal glands, which sit on top of the kidneys, help us deal with them. When we are under stress, our brain stimulates the pituitary gland to release a hormone that travels in the bloodstream to the adrenals. They, in turn, release other hormones, including adrenalin and cortisone, which give us temporary clarity and produce sugar to give us the strength we need to handle the stressful situation.

Our adrenal glands don't differentiate between various types of stress. Physical, emotional, environmental, mental, gravitational, chemical, thermal, nutritional—they're all treated similarly. Whether you're excited about vacation plans, won a lottery, or walked all day in shoes that were too tight, your adrenal glands are being affected. Too much stimulation over a period of time can weaken them and make it difficult for them to produce hormones.

Question 5: Stress on the adrenals causes more than general fatigue. It can cause slow pupil contraction, which lets in too much light, thereby making your eyes sensitive to light. If you always wear sunglasses, it may be a sign you're under too much stress. When you suddenly become dizzy after you stand up, either getting out of bed or while exercising, you may be responding to a drop in blood pressure, another response from tired adrenals.

Because muscles associated with the adrenal glands attach at the knees, a common but not widely known sign of overstress is knee pain or weak knees. Some of these muscles also hold the pelvis in place, so low back pain, especially in the sacroiliac area, can be a result of too much stress. If you are a runner or exercise vigorously and experience frequent knee or low back problems, make sure you're exercising properly and not overtraining or under too much stress.

Cortisol, produced by the adrenal glands, reduces inflammation from allergies. If you have allergies, your adrenal glands may be tired from secreting so much cortisol. Although there is no illness, the adrenal glands are overworked.

When adrenal glands are fatigued, the sodium balance in the body is disturbed. Hormones produced by the adrenals regulate your body's mineral balance. Sodium and potassium are regulated by one of these hormones, aldosterone. When your adrenal glands are fatigued, your body loses more sodium than usual and you may have a craving for salt. I'm not advocating you use more salt. Just be aware of the message: a craving for salty foods may be a sign of stress. Eliminating nutritional stress through the Anti-illness Diet is an excellent beginning to stress reduction.

Menopausal symptoms such as hot flashes, irritability, and weight gain can occur when the adrenals are too tired to produce hormones after the ovaries stop manufacturing them. This is a vital reason for women to strengthen their adrenal glands prior to menopause with diet, rest, exercise, and proper supplementation and to allow the body's natural functions to make the transition an easy one.

Perfectionists and workaholics tend to live stressful lives. These pressures may lead to tired adrenal glands and require the support of a balanced diet. It can be extremely stressful to try to follow every diet that seems to apply to you. Begin with the Anti-illness Diet in chapter 4, then incorporate the next most pertinent one. It is not necessary to follow any diet perfectly. Instead, make gradual changes in your eating habits and lifestyle. They will permanently affect your health and be more beneficial than would eating perfectly for a few weeks and months, then slipping back into old patterns that didn't work for you.

Question 6: Frequent headaches can come from a wide variety of sources, including food allergies, blood sugar irregularities, digestive problems, stress, alcohol, and caffeine. Keep this in mind as you follow your anti-illness program. Your headaches will disappear if they are related to the problems you are correcting through diet. If they persist, consult a doctor. Headaches can be signals for minor and major problems.

Frequent colds and flu can be a sign of a poor immune system. Although colds may be an inconvenience you have learned to live with, your immune system is your body's defense against major illnesses as well as minor ones. The Anti-illness Diet is the first step in building a strong immunity. For further recommendations, see the Strong Immune System Diet, chapter 5, which includes specific dietary supplements to strengthen your defense mechanisms.

You could feel generally run-down if your immune system is low, or from blood sugar imbalances. A low level of alcoholism (dependency on one or two drinks a day), food allergies, digestive problems, and infections, can all contribute to low immunity. Be aware of whether or not your run-down feeling is alleviated as you improve your nutritional program. It is likely you will see some improvement by the time you have been on the Anti-illness Diet a month or two. Some people report increased energy even sooner.

Swelling, bloating, and pains in the joints can be indicative of allergies, arthritis, premenstrual syndrome, or digestive problems. Again, you will often see improvements with the Anti-illness Diet alone, unless your pains and swelling are coming from other sources such as calcium deposits. If a good general diet is not sufficient to alleviate your symptoms, see the Arthritis Diet, chapter 5.

Eating disorders such as compulsive eating, bulimia, and anorexia are signaled by specific habits and attitudes around food. If you constantly diet even when everyone tells you you're thin enough, or if you feel heavy when the scales and people around you say you're not, you may be anorectic. Anorexia is not only an emotional problem, it also results in nutritional deficiences. If you've been hearing people tell you to gain weight, or if you think you can't be thin enough, do your body a favor and read the Anorexia Diet in chapter 5 (the ABCs of Eating).

Binging and purging (vomiting) is a sign of bulimia. Although there are similarities between bulimia and anorexia, each has differences explored in chapter 5. There are ways to stop this pattern if and when you are ready to do so, and there may be important consequences if you do not. The foods we eat provide us with necessary nutrients. In addition to not providing them, bulimia causes irritation to the stomach. Stop hurting your body and read the ABCs of Eating in chapter 5.

Compulsive eating is common to many women for physical and emotional reasons. Often, it is a result of an addiction or allergy to a specific food. A woman with a vaginal yeast infection like *Candida albicans* may crave bread, which contains yeast and will help the *Candida* flourish. Her body is addicted to whatever substances will keep the *Candida* active. Other health problems associated with compulsive eating include alcoholism, blood sugar imbalances, and some types of premenstrual syndrome. Allergies may be due to your body's inability to digest specific foods. For further help in the area of compulsive eating, see the Good Digestion Diet, the Candida Albicans Diet, the Blood Sugar Diet, and the Premenstrual Syndrome Diet, chapter 5. Emotional support is often beneficial, but finding and correcting the nutritional imbalances are essential for a permanent change.

YOUR REPRODUCTIVE SYSTEM

Premenstrual Syndrome (PMS):

    a. Do you presently use birth control pills? _____
       Have you used birth control pills in the past? _____ How long? _____
       Have your symptoms increased since then? _____

    b. Have you had a tubal ligation (tubes tied)? _____
       If yes, have your symptoms increased since then? _____

    c. During the first few days of your period, or prior to it, do you have:
       Menstrual cramps? _____
       Lower backache? _____
       Acne? _____

    d. Determining the presence of PMS and its severity:
       (This Menstrual Symptomology Questionnaire is reprinted with permission from Guy E. Abraham, M.D.)

       Grade your symptoms for your last menstrual cycle. If it was unusual, grade according to a typical cycle. Use the following key:

0 = none
1 = mild (symptoms present but do not interfere with activities)
2 = moderate (symptoms present and interfere, but you can function)
3 = severe (cannot function without medication, disabling)

Symptoms	Week Before	Week After Menses Ends
PMT-A		
Nervous tension	_____	_____
Mood swings	_____	_____
Irritability	_____	_____
Anxiety	_____	_____
	Total _____	Total _____
PMT-H		
Swelling of extremities	_____	_____
Weight gain (1 to 4 pounds)	_____	_____
Breast tenderness	_____	_____
Abdominal bloating	_____	_____
	Total _____	Total _____
PMT-C		
Headaches	_____	_____
Crave sweets	_____	_____
Increased appetite	_____	_____
Heart pounds	_____	_____
Fatigue	_____	_____
Dizziness or fainting	_____	_____
	Total _____	Total _____
PMT-D		
Depression	_____	_____
Forgetfulness	_____	_____
Crying	_____	_____
Confusion	_____	_____
Insomnia	_____	_____
	Total _____	Total _____
Add totals from each column	_____	_____

Candida albicans (a vaginal and/or systemic infection):
a. When do you remember feeling completely well? (approximate age or date)

_____

b. Do you have the following symptoms:
   Abdominal bloating _____   Fatigue _____
   Abnormal menstrual cycle __   Hives _____
   Anxiety _____   Increased premenstrual syndrome ____

Constipation _____   Loss of concentration _____
Crying _____   Loss of memory _____
Cystitis _____   Loss of self-confidence _____
Depression _____   Loss of sex drive _____
Diarrhea _____   Sensitivity to chemicals (food, perfume,
Endometriosis _____   cigarettes, and so on) _____
Excessive gas _____   Vaginal discharge _____
Extreme irritability _____ Vaginal itching _____

c. Did your symptoms begin with:
a chronic illness? _____
pregnancy? _____
birth control pills? _____
antibiotics? _____
eating a lot of sugar? _____

Cold Sores and Genital Herpes:

a. Do you get frequent or periodic cold sores in your mouth? _____

b. Do you have a profuse, watery vaginal discharge? _____

c. Do you have one or more sores on your vulva? _____

d. Is there burning on your vulva during urination? _____

e. Do any of these symptoms occur:
primarily under stress? _____
premenstrually? _____

Post-Menstrual Symptoms (Menopause and Osteoporosis):

a. How often do you have a period? _____

b. Are your periods regular or irregular? _____

c. How many days long is your cycle? _____

d. How long does the flow last? _____

e. Do you have hot flashes (sudden flash of heat, no sweating)? _____

f. Do you have increased facial hair? _____

g. Do you have increased vaginal dryness? _____

h. Do you have hot flushes (sweating, heat and redness on your chest and face, followed, occasionally, by coldness)? _____

i. Do you have backaches when you bend over? _____

j. Have you begun to notice arthritic-type pain? _____

k. Do you have blood relatives who have had
arthritis? _____
atherosclerosis? _____

osteoporosis? _____
leg cramps? _____

Amenorrhea (lack of menstruation):
When did you have your last period? _____

Do you exercise strenuously (run eight miles a day or more, do heavy weight training or aerobics for more than an hour a day, and so on)?

_____

Do you have very little total body fat? _____

Interpreting Your Reproductive System:

Premenstrual Syndrome (PMS). This is one name for a variety of complaints which occur from two weeks to a day before menses and usually stop when the menstrual flow begins or shortly thereafter. The work of gynecologist Dr. Guy Abraham is revolutionary in this area. He has classified PMS into types (PMT-A, PMT-H, PMT-C, and PMT-D), and has identified their specific causes and dietary and supplemental solutions. He estimated PMS was responsible for a $5-billion loss to American industries in 1956, and with more women in the work force today, he believes the present loss to be several times that amount. His findings have proven so successful in my own practice that many of the dietary changes mentioned in chapter 5 are taken directly from his fourteen years of research.

Both birth control pills and tubal ligation can cause hormonal changes that result in PMS or increase existing PMS symptoms. If your symptoms began or increased after either, the Premenstrual Syndrome Diet can help your body regain its balance. Progesterone therapy has been offered as an appropriate answer, but Dr. Abraham and many other gynecologists believe it is effective in only a small fraction of the cases, and progesterone worsens some symptoms of PMS. You may want to consider the noninvasive approach of dietary changes before introducing hormones into your system.

The Menstrual Symptomology Questionnaire will help you determine the presence of PMS and its severity. Specific diets and necessary nutrients for each type are discussed in detail in chapter 5. You may find you fall into more than one category. This is not unusual.

Although you may experience physical or emotional symptoms each month before you menstruate (and many women have both), to be considered PMS your symptoms must score as moderate to severe premenstrually. In addition, these symptoms must be mild or absent after your period begins.

	How to Tell the Severity of Your PMS		
Week Before Period	*Mild*	*Moderate*	*Severe*
PMT-A	less than 5	5–8	9–12
PMT-H	less than 5	5–8	9–12
PMT-C	less than 7	7–12	13–18
PMT-D	less than 6	6–10	11–15

Next, your score for the week *before* your period *must be greater than* the week after by the following amounts:

PMT-A	more than 4 points higher premenstrually
PMT-H	more than 4 points higher premenstrually
PMT-C	more than 6 points higher premenstrually
PMT-D	more than 5 points higher premenstrually

Example: If your score for PMT-A the week before your period is 7, and the week after is 1, you have PMT-A. The difference between the two scores is 6, which meets the criteria of being more than 4 points. If, on the other hand, you score 7 points the week before your period, and 5 points the week after, this is not considered PMS. Something else is going on. The difference between the two scores is only 2 points. You need a difference in this category of more than 4 points for your symptoms to be considered PMS.

Candida albicans. Vaginal infections can be caused by a fungus, protozoan, or bacteria. The most common type, *Candida albicans,* which can appear as vaginitis or have more widespread symptoms throughout your body, is caused by a fungus in the vagina and intestines and can be eradicated by nutritional means. Here, the helpful bacteria have been overrun by the *Candida* fungus and need to be reestablished in the vagina and intestines. If it looks as though *Candida* may be the source of your problems, see the Candida Albicans Diet in chapter 5 for nutritional solutions. This questionnaire helps identify the many symptoms of *Candida.* If you have vaginal infections that do not correlate with these questions, you may have one of the other two varieties of infections, both sexually transmitted. See your doctor or a nurse practitioner for an evaluation and treatment.

In many cases *Candida* infections are caused by large or repeated doses of antibiotics, which kill off the helpful bacteria and foster the growth of *Candida.* It can also begin with pregnancy or the use of birth control pills, which upset the hormone balance, or by a diet high in sugar, which feeds the fungus. *Candida* weakens the immune system, making it difficult for your body to fight off other illnesses.

Cold Sores and Genital Herpes. These related viruses seem to become more active with stress. If you have had herpes or cold sores, your body may always carry these viruses. Some amino acids (the components of proteins) common in food aggravate these conditions, while others alleviate them. The Herpes Diet in chapter 5 describes in detail the foods to avoid and those to eat and can help keep you free from symptoms. Reducing your dietary stress with the Anti-illness Diet can also be helpful in preventing a recurrence.

Post-Menstrual Symptoms. Many people consider these to be unavoidable. All of us go through menopause, and osteoporosis affects 90 percent of women over sixty. But menopausal symptoms are unnecessary, and the advances of osteoporosis can be slowed down or prevented.

Questions a through i relate to menopause. As we approach this natural change in our reproductive cycle, it is important to separate the avoidable from the unavoidable symptoms. It is natural, for instance, for the length and flow of our menstrual cycles to be reduced and eventually eliminated. Even vaginal dryness, indicative of hormonal changes, may be inevitable. But hot flashes and increased facial hair, hot flushes with sweating, and backaches may be eliminated if your adrenal glands can produce the hormones the reproductive system has stopped making. The Stressful Living Diet and the Menopause Diet, both in chapter 5, contain information on vitamin and mineral supplementation that can help ease this transition.

Questions j and k refer to osteoporosis, a reduction in bone density that often results in brittle bones. There is no definitive proof that it can be safely slowed down, stopped, or prevented. Estrogen therapy, a popular and effective solution, can cause cervical cancer. Mounting evidence indicates that osteoporosis is linked to the same calcium malabsorption problem that causes some forms of PMS. Dietary changes that help the calcium in your diet be absorbed into the bones and recommendations for weight-bearing exercise are all part of the Osteoporosis Diet found in chapter 5. If you are beginning to notice arthritic-type pains, or if you have relatives with signs of calcium imbalance such as arthritis, atherosclerosis, muscle cramps, or osteoporosis, you may want to incorporate the alterations suggested in the Osteoporosis Diet into your Anti-illness Diet as soon as possible for the greatest preventive care.

Amenorrhea. If you have amenorrhea, you do not menstruate. Amenorrhea may be due to excessively heavy exercise or very low body fat, or it may be due to other factors discussed in the Amenorrhea Diet in chapter 5. When exercise is reduced, or body fat is increased, menstruation often begins again. I have found some nutritional factors, based on Oriental medicine, to be quite effective in helping some women with amenorrhea begin menstruating again.

BEGIN PREVENTION THE ANTI-ILLNESS WAY

You have begun working with the first level of health: symptoms. What is more, with the help of your health diary, you have detected some causes for these symptoms. Now you're ready to move to the next level: prevention. A healthful diet with sufficient vitamins, minerals, and protein can prevent symptoms from recurring or occurring in the future. The next chapter presents a good, general nutritional program for all women. I call it the Anti-illness Diet. Although it is designed with women's health care in mind, it is a sound nutritional program that can benefit men and women alike.

The questionnaires in this chapter have directed you to specific diets for particular health problems, but before rushing to implement them, you need a solid nutritional foundation on which you can build. The Anti-illness Diet detailed in the following chapter is this foundation. Begin slowly with this basic diet and incorporate its principles into your life. If you find you want greater changes than it brings, you can integrate one or more of the specific diets found in chapter 5. Be patient. You are creating better eating habits that will last you the rest of your life.

CHAPTER FOUR
THE ANTI-ILLNESS DIET

My soul is dark with stormy riot,
Directly traceable to diet.
—SAMUEL HOFFENSTEIN

A HEALTHY DIET IS AN ANTI-ILLNESS DIET

An Anti-illness Diet consists primarily of whole, unprocessed foods. Furthermore, an Anti-illness Diet for women modifies the concept of whole foods to fit our nutritional needs and our ability to use nutrients throughout the various stages in our life. Whether you have a general feeling that your eating habits need to be improved or a specific health concern, the Anti-illness Diet will begin to ease your concern and begin to restore you to a higher level of health.

Following are all the components that make up the basic Anti-illness Diet. Unlike the diets many of us were raised on, it is significantly low in protein and fats and high in grains and legumes. Some of the factors that lead to many women's health problems, such as excessive amounts of dairy products, protein, sugar, and caffeine, are eliminated. The diet that remains will give you energy throughout the day and help you achieve your proper weight. It will give you an immediate feeling of better health and long-range protection. The Anti-illness Diet consists of the following food categories, in order of their importance and highest quantity:

Grains and legumes
Vegetables
Protein
Fruit
Nuts and seeds
Fats and oils

BEGIN WITH GRAINS AND LEGUMES

Too many women avoid eating whole grains and legumes (beans and peas) because they think these foods are fattening. Not so. Although they are dense foods, they are both low in fat and filling, so that eating a small amount is satisfying. Grains and legumes may be the key element lacking in your diet. They help balance your blood sugar level, whether yours is high, low, or "just right." They are high in fiber and provide bulk for healthy elimination. Most important, they contain an abundance of magnesium, the preventive mineral for such problems as premenstrual syndrome, osteoporosis, atherosclerosis, and arthritis. Figure 4–1 shows the amount of calcium and magnesium in grains, as well as in other foods that can be part of your Anti-illness Diet.

Figure 4–1 Calcium and Magnesium in Common Foods
A list of foods to include in your diet that contain both calcium and magnesium.
Taken from *Nutrition Almanac*

FOOD	AMOUNT	CALCIUM/mg	MAGNESIUM/mg
Bran, wheat	½ cup	33.9	139.5
Cornmeal	½ cup	10	62.5
Millet, dry	½ cup	22.8	184.5
Oatmeal, cooked	½ cup	11	25
Brown rice, cooked	½ cup	9	22.5
Haddock	½ pound	52	54.5
Red snapper	½ pound	36.50	63.50
Almonds, raw	½ cup	166	193
Tofu	⅕ pound	128	111
Tomato, raw	1 medium	20	21
Tomato juice	1 cup	17	20

Today we eat only *half* as much grain as our ancestors did around the turn of the century, and most of it is refined. Some researchers are convinced this reduction in whole grains is responsible for many of our current illnesses. Grains are more than whole wheat bread. They include all forms of wheat, rye, oats (as in oatmeal), cornmeal, brown rice, barley, millet, buckwheat, and triticale. They come in the form of whole grains (sometimes called "groats"), cracked grain, flakes, and flours.

Wheat is our most common grain, and we eat much of it as refined flour in breads, baked goods, crackers, pasta, and breakfast cereals. Almost all commercially available foods made from grains, such as rye bread and buckwheat pancake mix, are made from enriched white flour with small amounts of other grains added for taste and are missing the vitamins and minerals you need to be healthy. It's not difficult to find whole grain baked goods, crackers, pasta, and cereals in most supermarkets if you read labels carefully. But you will find a larger selection in health food stores, where you can also buy whole wheat flour to make some of your own baked goods. Other forms of wheat, such as bulgur (partially cooked cracked whole wheat) and wheat berries can be found in these and other specialty stores. If you're feeling adventuresome, ask or look for directions on how to prepare them. Quite simply, they're all nutritious forms of wheat. Wheat germ, although high in B vitamins, vitamin E, protein, and the essential fatty acids a woman's body needs so much, tends to get rancid quickly, and rancid foods can be carcinogenic. In my opinion, it's much easier to get wheat germ with the rest of the wheat and bran in the form of whole wheat products. I've tried wheat germ in all forms and packaging, including raw wheat germ vacuum-packed in tins, and all of it tastes rancid.

Brown rice is probably the next most familiar whole grain. Brown rice is more filling than white rice and has a slightly nutty flavor. It takes a little longer to cook but otherwise is prepared essentially the same as white rice. Brown rice crackers and rice cakes, which are thick, light, and crunchy with a flavor like popcorn, are available in health food stores and a few supermarkets. Brown rice flour can be substituted in small amounts for other flours in baked goods. It is lighter and less sticky than wheat or oats, and gives cakes, cookies, and bread the delicate consistency of fine white flour. Brown rice is a good alternative for people with a sensitivity to wheat and makes a nice change in its various forms.

Buckwheat, or kasha, is not from the wheat family, so people with a wheat sensitivity *can* eat buckwheat. It can be used in place of rice or millet as a side dish or as a breakfast food. Kasha is a staple grain in Jewish cooking, and the basis for soba, or buckwheat, noodles, a popular Japanese dish. Most soba found in Oriental markets and health food stores contain some wheat, but there is a 100 percent buckwheat noodle available for people who need or want to avoid wheat. Whether you serve buckwheat instead of rice, or use buckwheat noodles in pasta dishes, try including this nutritious grain in your diet.

Oats are most often consumed in oatmeal, oatmeal cookies, and granola cereal. Oatmeal is one of the best cereals you can eat; it has been found to lower cholesterol and is soothing to the colon. Oatmeal cookies, especially when they are made with whole wheat flour, are a nutritious snack, but commercial granola, even the health food varieties, is usually so heavily sweetened it is best mixed with other, less-sweet cereals, or made without so much honey. Recipes for easy-to-prepare granolas can be found in *The Deaf Smith Country Cookbook* (see References following Afterword). Oat bran, tastier and less fibrous than wheat bran, is also being used to lower cholesterol, as it helps the body excrete cholesterol in larger amounts. All high-fiber grains increase cholesterol elimination by triggering the liver into converting it into bile acids, which the body quickly eliminates. Oat bran can be used as a cereal or to make muffins. Instead of always reaching for wheat, explore the light, distinctive taste of oats.

Corn is both a grain and a vegetable. Dried and ground into meal, it is a grain; fresh corn is a vegetable. Cornmeal is used in muffins, tortillas, and corn chips and can be added to pancake mix. Many commercial brands of corn chips are high in oils and salt, although it is possible to find more healthful ones in health food stores. Eat even these kinds only in small quantities. Popcorn, an old favorite, is another form of this grain. It acts as a scrub brush in the intestines and provides an excellent form of fiber. In excess, it can be an irritant, so chew it well and don't eat more than a few cups at a time.

Barley is most often added to soups, although it can also be served as a side dish. Cook it alone, with sautéed mushrooms, or with brown rice (add rice a half hour after the barley has been simmering so they are both ready at the same time). Like oatmeal, barley is very soothing and easy to digest. When I counsel patients with digestive problems, colitis, or other internal irritations, I frequently suggest they incorporate barley into their diet. There is no reason why this soup thickener should be eaten so infrequently or be limited only to soups.

Rye's distinct flavor is a little heavy for some people used to refined wheat products and the mild taste of rye bread. It is only a minor ingredient in commercial rye bread, but you can find 100 percent rye bread in some stores made with a light-tasting, light rye flour, which is a good alternative if you have a wheat sensitivity. Both dark and light rye flours are available—the dark being more distinct in flavor, the light having a milder taste. This grain is most commonly found in rye crackers. Rye flakes, another health food store item, can be added to a homemade granola or cooked into a hot cereal. A few commercial hot cereals already contain rye, which provides a variety from the old standby wheat. I often add a little rye flour to pancakes and muffins for a change of taste.

Millet is a grain traditionally used in Africa, Asia, and parts of the Middle East. A mild grain that cooks like rice, hulled millet has a slightly sweet, nutty flavor. It is the most alkaline of all grains and is easily digested. Use it in soups, as a hot cereal, or in place of rice as a side dish or in recipes that call for rice. Millet meal or millet flour, ground in a little seed grinder, can be added to recipes for muffins or pancakes.

Triticale is a new grain developed by crossing wheat and rye and is higher in protein than other grains. The sweet taste of triticale is found in some breads and cereals in health food stores. You can use it whole or flaked in cereals or as flour in breads and cookies. Since it is low in gluten (high-gluten grains are sticky and hold baked goods together well), mix triticale with such glutinous grains as wheat or oats for baking.

Legumes include all kinds of peas (black-eyed, green, split) and beans (garbanzo, pinto, kidney, azuki, soy, lima, black, white, red, and mung), as well as lentils, tofu, and peanuts. They are all high in iron and some of the B vitamins. Menstruating or pregnant women, whose need for iron increases at these times, should be consuming these iron-rich foods. They are also ideal foods for anyone with a blood sugar problem since they turn into sugar slowly and provide sustained energy and support. They're inexpensive, filling additions to your diet. Added to soup, made into dips, or mixed with grains to make a complete protein, legumes are an important food for healthy people.

If they tend to give you gas, begin with a small, well-cooked quantity and allow your body to adjust to them. Cook them slowly over a low heat to make them more easily digested.

Peanuts, including peanut butter, are an exception in this category of desirable foods because they are extremely difficult to digest and high in peanut oil, which has been recently linked to coronary heart disease. One report, published in the *International Clinical Nutrition Review*, indicated that 90 percent of monkeys, rats, and rabbits on a cholesterol free diet developed atherosclerosis when peanut oil was added to their food. If you insist on eating peanuts, eat them infrequently, and only if your cholesterol is normal and you have no digestive problems.

EAT A LOT OF FRESH VEGETABLES

A high-vegetable diet is an "anticonstipation" diet, since vegetables provide both fiber and water. It is also an "anti-colon-cancer" diet, because the bulk it provides reduces the time your intestinal bacteria need to convert bile acids into carcinogens. Historically, cultures with high-fiber diets have low levels of colon cancer, and both whole grains and fresh vegetables are high in fiber.

Fresh vegetables are also excellent sources of vitamins and minerals. Dark green leafy vegetables, including broccoli, are particularly high in vitamin A, which is needed for a healthy liver and clear skin, and is helpful to the eyes. Other vegetables are high in important trace minerals. Begin to eat a wider variety of vegetables of all colors: yellow, orange, dark green, red, and white, and rotate them to keep from eating the same ones over and over. To give you an idea of the selection available, and help you broaden your experience of this important food group, choose from the following:

alfalfa sprouts, artichokes, bean sprouts, beets, beet greens, bell peppers (green and sweet red), bok choy, brussel sprouts, cabbage, carrots, cauliflower, celery, chinese cabbage, chinese snow peas, collard greens, corn, crookneck squash, cucumbers, eggplant, jerusalem artichokes, jícama, leeks, lettuce (except iceberg), mushrooms, okra, onions, parsley, parsnips, peas, potatoes, radishes, spinach, string beans, summer squash, sweet potatoes, tomatoes, turnips, turnip greens, winter squash, yams, and zucchini—to name some of the most common.

Fresh vegetables are better for you than frozen, and I recommend you avoid canned vegetables, which are overcooked and contain high amounts of sodium. Frozen vegetables are not much better. For example, frozen green peas have a bright, uniform color because they are washed in a chemical solution of EDTA, which removes important minerals from the surface of many vegetables and reduces the level of trace minerals in our bodies as well. Eating frozen vegetables constantly can deplete your body rather than add to your health.

Eat fresh vegetables in season whenever possible. To retain as much of their nutrients as you can, and to unlock those trapped in the fiber, cook them very lightly and chew them well. Steaming and stir-frying in a little vegetable oil are the most healthful ways to cook them.

The only fresh vegetable to avoid is iceburg lettuce, sometimes called head lettuce. This pale lettuce contains more water than vitamins and seems to relax the colon, lengthening the time it takes for wastes to be eliminated. Instead, try raw spinach, which has more vitamins and stimulates the action of the bowels, in salads, or use butter lettuce, red leaf, endive, or romaine.

PROTEINS, OUR OVERRATED STAPLES

Animal proteins contain all the necessary amino acids needed to build and maintain muscles and other tissues and to help produce hormones. Plant proteins (beans, peas, grains, nuts, and seeds) need to be combined to make complete proteins. However, Frances Moore Lappé, author of *Diet for a Small Planet* and *Recipes for a Small Planet*, two books on vegetarian eating and protein combining, recently announced in an article in the *Whole Life Times*, a national health magazine, that incomplete proteins combine in our bodies and we do not have to be concerned about mixing them to get sufficient protein. In fact, if you're eating a well-balanced diet such as the Anti-illness Diet, you can't help but get enough protein.

Most of us eat too much. We've been raised on a high-protein diet, often eating meat or other proteins at each meal. Eggs, yogurt, or cereal with milk (which makes a combined protein) are typical breakfast foods; lunch often consists of a cheese or meat sandwich, or cottage cheese; dinner is usually our main meal, with meat, chicken, or fish, vegetables, and a starch. Three generous helpings of protein a day adds fat and density to our diet rather than fiber. Because it's filling and satisfying, it takes the place of other satisfying, filling foods—the grains and legumes we need for better health.

Like calcium, the quality of protein is more crucial than quantity. Eating too many foods high in protein can trigger malabsorption problems and produce excess waste products that overload the colon and kidneys and can cause fluid imbalance and edema.

Excess protein contributes to aging, cancer, atherosclerosis, kidney disease, digestive problems, premenstrual syndrome, and arthritis. It adds saturated fats to a diet that *must* be low in fats if we are going to reduce our risk of breast and ovarian cancer. It decreases the production of prostaglandins (chemicals that regulate cell function and control calcium movement) in the pancreas and central nervous system, which can lead to premenstrual sugar cravings, overeating, and hypoglycemic reactions. This last fact is interesting, for in 1936, high-protein diets were advocated for treating hypoglycemia. Recent research has shown that hypoglycemic blood sugar levels respond more favorably to a diet high in complex carbohydrates, and low in protein intake, which releases sugar slowly and consistently into the bloodstream and contains fewer wastes to stress the kidneys, bladder, and colon.

We must reduce our total protein intake if we are going to be healthy, and much of the protein we eliminate should be animal protein. The animal proteins you do eat should be low in fats: fish, poultry without the skin, and small amounts of low-fat or nonfat dairy products for those who can tolerate them, like low-fat milk, nonfat yogurt, and mozzarella cheese. Since eggs are high in fat, eat them sparingly, rather than daily. All fish that swim are good sources of protein, but shellfish, which are scavengers, are toxic from eating debris at the bottom of the ocean and high in fat. Eat them very infrequently if at all.

For women, even those on a vigorous exercise program, one or two small helpings of protein a day is usually sufficient. If you eat a healthy diet you don't have to concentrate on getting enough protein, even if you are a vegetarian. All proteins are made from amino acids, which provide us with building blocks for healthy muscle, hormones, and other tissues. Our body knows how to manufacture some of these amino acids, but it can't make eight of them, called "essential amino acids." These must come from our foods. Animal protein has all of them, while grains, nuts, seeds, and legumes contain some, but not all.

Grains, nuts, and seeds, when combined with legumes, will give you complete high-quality proteins. Soy milk, tofu (soybean curd used in Oriental cooking), and soy-based protein powders are good alternatives for people who want less animal protein in their diet. Added to a diet low in animal protein, they improve your nutritional program; however, if you are a vegetarian, you need to be attentive to potential deficiencies. Plant proteins lack vitamin B_{12}, necessary for protein, fat, and carbohydrate metabolism. A deficiency in B_{12} can lead to a form of anemia that is often masked by folic acid, found in abundance in green leafy vegetables. If you are a strict vegetarian, you may need to take a vitamin B_{12} supplement. Grains and legumes also can cause a zinc deficiency, since the phytates they contain do not permit zinc absorption. One signal of a zinc deficiency is light-headedness. This is not the result of a pure diet, but a lack of zinc. Vegetarians would be wise to add zinc to their diet for added insurance. However, large quantities of zinc can pull copper out of your body, so zinc supplements should be taken with caution and preferably with small amounts of copper added.

Vegetarianism can be a healthy dietary alternative if you:

1. Combine proteins properly.
2. Take a vitamin B_{12} supplement.
3. Take a zinc supplement.
4. Eat whole foods low in refined sugar.

DON'T FORGET FRESH FRUIT

In addition to contributing fiber to our diet, fruit is an excellent intestinal cleanser. Although it is an important component in your diet, it is also high in fructose, which is a natural sugar. If you have high or low blood sugar or bloat premenstrually, eating a lot of fruit can cause some of the same problems as eating sugar or honey. Studies have also shown that some people have as much sensitivity to fructose as others have to refined sugar. According to biochemist Roger J. Williams, this sensitivity is increased in people with high cholesterol levels. If you have high cholesterol, fatigue, hypoglycemia, or diabetes, a large fruit salad for lunch or large quantities of fruit throughout the day is not wise. In fact, a lot of fructose in any form can be counterproductive to a healthy diet. Biochemist Jeffrey Bland points out that chemically, fructose is as much a simple sugar as sucrose and will have the same kind of metabolic side effects.

When eaten with other foods, the sugar in fruit combines with proteins and grains and begins to ferment into alcohol in your colon, causing gas and cramping. For easier digestion, eat your fruit as a snack rather than with meals. If you want fresh fruit for dessert, wait half an hour or more before eating it.

Whole fruit contains all the available nutrients, while juices are higher in fructose and lower in fiber, and don't retain many of the vitamins and minerals stored just under the fruit's skin. It can take six to ten oranges to make an eight-ounce glass of orange juice. That's a lot of sugar! If you want fruit juice occasionally, drink small amounts and dilute it with one-third water or with a little sparkling mineral water.

NUTS AND SEEDS, THE EASY-TO-CARRY SNACK

Most nuts and seeds are high in magnesium, some contain calcium, and all are rich in trace minerals. They are packed with protein, B vitamins, and essential fatty acids. They're also high in fats, both a plus and a minus: they take longer to digest, which gives you the advantage of feeling full longer, but in substantial amounts they increase your fat intake and add unwanted weight. If you can control the amount you eat, small quantities make excellent snacks and take up very little space in your purse.

Because of their fat and protein content, nuts are difficult to digest, so get into the habit of chewing them very well. Sesame seeds are tiny as well, so make sure you chew them thoroughly to break down their outer covering and prevent them from passing through your intestines untouched and undigested. The wide variety of nuts and seeds to choose from includes: almonds, brazil nuts, cashews, hazelnuts, macadamias, pecans, pine nuts, pistachios (unsalted and undyed), pumpkin seeds, sesame seeds, sunflower seeds, and walnuts.

Unshelled raw nuts and seeds remain fresh longest, and almonds are lowest in fats. Next best are shelled raw nuts and seeds. Roasted, they are more likely to become rancid, since heat contributes to the oxidation of the natural oils and contributes to spoilage.

FATS AND OILS, IMPORTANT IN SMALL QUANTITIES

Although we've been told to avoid fats for weight control and to prevent health problems such as breast cancer, we do need to include some unsaturated fats in our diet. Polyunsaturated vegetable oils, in the form of cold-pressed safflower, corn, sesame, soy, and sunflower oils, are the best source because they are high in essential fatty acids.

Prostaglandins are chemicals that regulate cell function and control the movement of calcium and the activities of many enzymes. They are short lived and must constantly be replaced. One major function of EFAs is to provide the raw materials needed to make prostaglandins. The Pritikin Diet advocates no fats or oils for some people, but this can be dangerous, since

A lack of EFAs can cause:

hair loss

eczema

a poor immune system

infertility

a fatty liver

poor healing from cuts and wounds

A lack of EFAs has been linked to arthritis, cancer, cataracts, skin diseases, heart diseases, arteriosclerosis, and menstrual problems. Our body cannot manufacture EFAs, so we must obtain them from our foods. You want some, in the form of vegetable oils, in your diet each day. Cold-pressed safflower oil, highest in EFAs, can be used in salad dressing to give you most of what you need. Oils which are not cold-pressed have been exposed to heat, and heating destroys essential fatty acids.

Animal fats are saturated and contain no EFAs. It is best to eat less or eliminate them to reduce your total fat intake. It's the high *total* fat content that is implicated in many serious illnesses. If you don't want to give up butter entirely, you can cut its saturation in half by following the recipe for a spread called Better Butter in this chapter. Margarine is no solution to the problem of saturated fats (see What's Wrong with How We Eat? later in this chapter), but Better Butter can give you the advantages of vegetable oils with the taste of butter.

A PRACTICAL GUIDE TO ANTI-ILLNESS EATING

Now that you know something about the foods and food groups that make up the Anti-illness Diet, we'll take a step-by-step look at each meal, with suggestions for easy preparation.

BREAKFAST, THE FORGOTTEN MEAL

Although almost everybody knows bodies need some nourishment in the morning, many people still don't eat breakfast. Either they are not hungry when they first get up, believe breakfast gives them an increased appetite the rest of the day, or say they don't have time to prepare it. It's important to give your body some food in the morning to help stabilize your energy and provide needed nutrients, so eat breakfast every morning, even if you don't eat much. It may appear to give you an increased appetite at first, but the hunger is a signal your body desperately needs fuel. If this sudden appetite concerns you, divide the same amount of food you've been eating for two meals into three. In a short time, you'll adapt to three meals with no additional hunger. Choose meals that are quick to prepare, or get up fifteen minutes earlier, but make time to give yourself the foods you need before rushing into the day's activities. If you happen to enjoy a large breakfast, eat wholesome foods. Turn your breakfast calories into health, rather than eating refined empty calories.

Some people like protein for breakfast, others prefer complex carbohydrates (whole grains), or fruit. Find which is the most satisfying for you. If you don't like traditional breakfast foods, experiment with some that may seem unusual to eat for breakfast. Leftovers from dinner, like spaghetti or chili, may be more appealing to you than eggs or cereal. Go ahead and eat them as long as the pasta is made from whole grains and the chili is low in animal fat.

If you buy your baked products, look for bread or muffins *without* enriched flour, sugar, or a lot of fats. Read the labels carefully until you know which brands are best. Homemade muffins take very little time to put together and make delicious additions to a meal or can be a light, portable breakfast. Muffin mixes from health food stores are usually made from whole grains, without added sweeteners, while those in supermarkets often contain enriched flours and sugar. Pancake mixes are the same, so get yours from a health food store or make your own. Oats can be easily ground into flour in a blender. Since they are mucilaginous (sticky), they work well in pancakes and muffins.

If you prefer cereal, find one with very little sugar or honey. Granolas usually contain a lot of sugar or honey and are frequently made with coconut or palm kernel oils—the two you want most to avoid. The less processed the cereal, the better it is for you, which is why oatmeal ranks high on the list of good breakfast foods. Cooked with a little diluted apple juice, it is naturally sweet and needs no added milk. Other hot cereals made from whole grains and cold cereals with a low sugar content, like Grape Nuts, Grape Nuts Flakes, Shredded Wheat, Nutri-Grain, and Special K, provide a wide variety to choose from. If you have a dairy sensitivity or would like to decrease your dairy intake, use soy milk on your cereals, in pancakes, and in all baked goods. It tastes a little different than milk, but many people quickly develop a taste for it. I've been using soy milk for years and now prefer its taste to cow's milk.

If you eat eggs, they can be prepared without butter by poaching, boiling, or cooking them in non-stick pans. Avoid Teflon, which can scrape off and allow the aluminum underneath to get into your food (aluminum toxicity has been linked to Alzheimer's disease). If you want an omelet, make one with vegetables rather than cheese.

Protein drinks are a quick solution for women who either are busy in the morning or want a light meal. Read the labels of commercial protein powders carefully and select a soy-based rather than a milk-based powder to avoid a calcium imbalance. Soy contains both calcium and magnesium. Some protein powders list fructose, sucrose, or other sugars as one of the first three ingredients. That means it's too sweet for health-conscious people. Find one with little or no sweetener and add a piece of fruit or one-quarter cup of fruit juice, instead. If you like, you can make your own protein drink with the recipe given later in the chapter.

STOP FOR LUNCH

By the middle of the day your body should be ready to stop for lunch. Give it a rest while you refuel. If you can fit it into your lifestyle, and if it feels comfortable, make lunch your main meal. A small amount of protein eaten at this time will give you energy in the afternoon. Protein takes four or five hours to digest, which makes lunch a better time to eat it than dinner. Because you need both fiber and the nutrients they contain, vegetables should be included at lunch and dinner. What you eat and how relaxed you are when you have your meal can influence how you feel the rest of the day, so make time for lunch. Eat it slowly, even if you only have a few minutes. Be calm; chew your food well. Don't eat in your car, while doing housework, or while you're working at your desk.

You can bring a variety of foods from home for lunch, including last night's leftovers, or find somewhere to eat where the choices will fit into your Anti-illness Diet. The food at fast-food restaurants is rarely of high quality, except for the salad bars at some, and even then many of the vegetables are washed in chemicals to keep them looking fresh longer. If money is a concern, bring your lunch and give yourself a high-quality meal.

UNWIND WITH DINNER

The ideal dinner is a meal of complex carbohydrates and vegetables. The starches in beans, grains, and starchy vegetables are filling and satisfying. They will keep your blood sugar level during the rest of the evening, and you'll be less likely to want something sweet later. If you do have protein for dinner, be kind to your digestive system and keep the amount small. Concentrate on whatever grains and vegetables are available. Be conscious and do your best.

If your family insists on dinners complete with protein, and you don't want to fix separate meals for yourself, eat a small portion and save the rest for your lunch the following day—or eat everything except the protein. Whole grain noodles or whole grains, such as brown rice, millet, buckwheat, and barley, are simple to fix if you want to add a substantial dish to the family table. Many of them can be reheated, so there's no need to cook them every day.

Dining out, whether in restaurants or at friends' homes, can be difficult at first. Many foods, while not ideal, are acceptable if you only have them occasionally. White rice, white bread, and white pasta are examples. Don't make an entire meal of them, but a little of anything with enough vegetables (cooked or in a salad) can get you through almost any meal. Most often, vegetables and either a potato or another starch can be ordered. Fish or chicken are standard fare in enough restaurants that you shouldn't have to go hungry or off your program.

WHEN IT'S SNACK TIME, KEEP IT HEALTHY

Many people can eat almost anything occasionally, but if your snacks are filled with fat and sugar like ice cream, pastry, and candy, you're defeating yourself. They promote illness, not health. Instead of feeling guilty after succumbing to them, or deprived, find snacks that taste good and are filling. Homemade cookies and cakes made with whole grains and low quantities of sweeteners are an excellent alternative to bakery goods. Or try whole grain crackers or hot-air popped popcorn, which you can turn into Popcorn Supreme (see recipe section in this chapter). If you must have dessert, have one or two bites, or share a portion with a friend, rather than eat it all.

A WORD ABOUT BEVERAGES

Water is the best beverage you can drink, at the rate of half a glass an hour whenever you remember. In its pure form it is an excellent cleanser. But don't drink it or any other liquid with your meals since they dilute your stomach acids and make it harder to digest your food. While water is the best liquid, other beverages, like mineral water and herb teas, are fine. Decaffeinated coffee is better than caffeinated, and a glass of wine from time to time is better than two or three, or daily drinking. Coffee substitutes made from roasted grains, like Caffix and Postum (which don't always taste like coffee but have a heartiness reminiscent of coffee), are good alternatives to black coffee or tea if you like a more substantial hot beverage than herb tea.

AND ONE ABOUT COOKING UTENSILS

While there is not enough space to devote to cooking utensils in this book, it is important to address the problem of cooking with aluminum pots and pans. The acids in some foods dissolve minute quantities of aluminum into the foods we eat. Aluminum is toxic to the central nervous system and has been strongly implicated in Parkinson's disease, Alzheimer's disease, dementia, and poor memory in studies published in the *Lancet* and the *New England Journal of Medicine*. It is of particular interest to women that aluminum tends to lodge in our bones, preventing the absorption of calcium, and can thus be a factor in osteoporosis.

The safest cookware you can use is enamel-coated aluminum or steel, which should be discarded when scratches permeate the metal, and glass. Stainless steel is acceptable, and ironware can actually be beneficial by releasing small quantities of iron into the bloodstream which can help prevent iron anemia.

SPECIFIC SUGGESTIONS FOR MEALS

Recipes for asterisked items appear in the following section.

BREAKFAST

Eating Breakfast at Home

Whole grain toast or muffins with *Better Butter or apple butter
*Whole Grain Pancakes with a little pure maple syrup, unsweetened apple-
sauce, or jam made with pure fruit (no honey or sugar)
A poached or boiled egg with toast or muffin
Scrambled egg with sautéed onions and mushrooms
Cold cereal with *Soy Milk or low-fat milk
*Oatmeal with Apple Juice
*Millet with Raisins and Almonds
Rice cakes with almond butter
A piece of fruit
Baked yam (cook it while you're dressing)

*Do-It-Yourself Protein Drink
Occasionally, unsweetened yogurt with fruit or cereal

Eating Breakfast Out

Oatmeal with low-fat milk or apple juice
Omelet (spinach and mushroom, sautéed vegetable, ratatouille, Spanish)
Grape Nuts or other low-sugar cereal with low-fat milk
Fruit
Bran muffin (usually too sweet, but an emergency breakfast with some beneficial ingredients)

LUNCH

Eating Lunch at Home or Bringing It to Work

Salad with beans (pinto, red, garbanzo) and whole grain roll
Salad with a small amount of chicken, turkey, tuna, egg, or sardines
Salad with a little low-fat cheese (a nice occasional treat)
A hearty soup, like lentil or bean, with whole grain crackers and a salad
*Vegetable Slaw with chicken on corn tortilla
Chicken breast and marinated vegetables
Steamed or sautéed vegetables with brown rice or millet
*Pasta Primavera (cold pasta salad)
*Hummus (garbanzo bean dip) with whole grain crackers and salad
*Tabbouli (cold cracked wheat salad) and *Hummus with raw vegetables
Occasionally, cottage cheese and raw vegetables

Eating Lunch Out

Salad with tuna, egg, or chicken
Salad bar with bean salad and/or garbanzo beans, and bread or crackers (a little cheese occasionally)
Chicken or fish with salad or cooked vegetables
Tuna, chicken, turkey, or egg-salad sandwich with coleslaw (get the best bread available)
Soup, salad, and a roll or crackers (you can always bring crackers)
Chinese vegetables with chicken and a little rice
Vegetable omelet with roll or crackers

DINNER

Eating Dinner at Home

*Spicy Chinese Vegetables and Soba Noodles
Sautéed vegetables with brown rice, kasha, or baked potato
Steamed vegetables with millet or brown rice
Lentil and barley soup with salad
Whole grain pasta with marinara sauce and salad

*Chicken Breasts in Wine and Tamari Sauce
Broiled fish or chicken with salad or vegetables
Curried vegetables with tofu and brown rice
Vegetable soup with whole grain noodles or rye crackers
Corn tortillas with beans and hot sauce (salsa), and salad
Corn bread and baked beans with salad
Spanish rice with vegetables or salad
Whole grain pasta with steamed vegetables and tomato sauce
Salad and baked potato

Eating Dinner Out

Broiled fish or chicken with vegetables and salad
Chicken or fish dishes with sauces on the side (use sparingly), with vegetables and salad
Chinese food with chicken or bean curd (tofu) and a little rice (no pork or shrimp)
Italian food: veal, chicken, or fish, with salad and side of pasta
Chicken enchilada or chicken tostada (no cheese) with salsa
Soup and salad

And Occasionally:

Pizza (with mushrooms, green peppers, onions, olives) and salad
Spaghetti (with tomato-based sauce)
Lean beef or veal entrée with salad and vegetables
Almost anything in moderation

SNACKS

At Home or Out

Homemade cookies using maple syrup and whole grains
Whole grain bran or corn muffins with *Better Butter
Nuts and seeds (eight to twelve nuts, small handful of seeds)
Small amounts of dried apples, apricots, figs, or pears (two to four pieces, since they're high in fructose)
Whole grain crackers with nut butter (almond, cashew, and so on)
Corn chips made with safflower or other acceptable oil (a few)
Whole wheat pretzels with sesame seeds instead of salt
*Popcorn Supreme
Cold sliced yam
Raw vegetables
Fruit

Beverages

Water with a little fresh lemon juice
Mineral water with lemon juice or a little fruit juice
Herb teas, hot or iced (sweetened with licorice root)
Coffee substitutes: Postum, Caffix, Pioneer, and so on
Decaffeinated coffee (Swiss, or water processed, whenever possible)

ANTI-ILLNESS RECIPES

BETTER BUTTER

For those of you who are not ready to give up the taste of butter, this is an excellent way to reduce your saturated fats. It combines the saturated fats in butter with the polyunsaturated fats in safflower oil. By using cold-pressed oil, you are giving yourself the essential fatty acids our bodies need so much. If you eat the same amount of Better Butter as plain butter, you're cutting your saturated fat intake in half.

¼ pound butter at room temperature

½ cup cold-pressed safflower oil

Blend with a fork and refrigerate.
Makes ½ pound.

WHOLE GRAIN PANCAKES

These pancakes are wheat free and can be made with a variety of grains. One grain should be sticky, such as oats. You can change the recipe by adding millet or buckwheat, ground into flour in a small seed grinder, a little rye flour, or anything else that happens to be around. A few whole grain pancakes in the morning makes a delicious breakfast of unforbidden food. They contain no added fats and, if you eat them with a little unsweetened jam or a few tablespoons of pure maple syrup, are no different than eating toast. However, the psychological freedom that comes from eating pancakes can be exhilarating to someone who is used to dieting.

Mix together

2 cups of whole grain flours (either the ones suggested here or your variations):

1 cup corn meal

½ cup brown rice flour (available at health food store)

½ cup oat flour (grind oatmeal in blender)

Add:

1½ cups of low-fat milk or soy milk

1 egg, or equivalent amount of egg replacer (found in health food store)

½ teaspoon baking powder (use Rumford brand or other brand without aluminum)

Serves a hungry family of four. Save any leftover batter in the refrigerator for another breakfast.

SOY MILK

When you want to cut back on dairy products to prevent calcium overkill or because of a dairy sensitivity, soy milk is an excellent substitute both in cooking and with cereal. If you are using it exclusively for cooking you may want to eliminate the honey, which is added only for taste. You can make a large batch of soy milk and freeze the extra in plastic or glass jars, being careful not to fill the container to the top to prevent breaking the container.

Place 1 pound of dry soy beans in a large jar or bowl (larger than a quart). Soak in water for one to three days in refrigerator to prevent sprouting.

Combine 1 cup of soaked beans and 1 quart water in blender and mix until fine. Strain into pot through cheesecloth.

Bring to boil and cook at low flame 20 to 30 minutes (the longer it cooks, the thicker it becomes).

Skim, and strain through strainer.

Repeat with remaining beans.

Add 1 tablespoon honey or pure maple syrup for each 1½ quarts.

Makes 6 quarts.

OATMEAL WITH APPLE JUICE

Try this if you like hot cereal and want to avoid both cow's milk and soy milk. It is a presweetened, moist cereal without sugar or honey that cooks while you're dressing in the morning. Nothing could be simpler to prepare or more beneficial to help eliminate cholesterol buildup, keep blood sugar level, and provide natural fiber. Besides, it tastes good.

¼ to ½ cup of dry rolled oats (oatmeal)

Cover with apple juice diluted by half with water.

Bring to boil and simmer, covered, 5 to 10 minutes.

Add more juice if additional moisture or sweetener is desired.

Makes one serving.

MILLET WITH RAISINS AND ALMONDS

This combination of fruit, grain, and nuts ought to be difficult to digest but is not. When cooked, both the raisins and nuts become more digestible. Serve it as is, with low-fat milk or soy milk, or with a teaspoon of cold-pressed safflower oil and a little tamari sauce (high-quality soy sauce). The blend of sweet and salt is a pleasant surprise. If this amount is too much for one meal, save it and reheat for another.

Bring to a boil and simmer, covered, 20 to 30 minutes or until millet is tender:

½ cup millet

1 cup water

1 tablespoon raisins

6 to 8 almonds

Makes two servings.

DO-IT-YOURSELF PROTEIN DRINK

Germinated seeds and nuts are added to soy protein for this variation of the standard protein-powder-and-juice drink. To germinate, simply soak the nuts and seeds overnight. Their protein content is increased and their fat content decreased through germination. Rinse and refrigerate any extra to be used later in the week. The refrigerated nuts and seeds should be rinsed once a day to keep them fresh. Soy milk or tofu can be used in place of more expensive protein powder, which often contains unwanted sugar.

Blend together:

½ cup soy milk or ⅙ pound tofu

¼ cup apple juice

½ cup berries or ½ piece of fruit (banana, peach, or other)

6 germinated almonds

1 tablespoon germinated sunflower seeds

Makes one serving.

For added B vitamins and energy, add brewer's yeast powder or flakes. Begin with ½ teaspoon and gradually build up to 2 tablespoons. If you begin with too much at first, you could get gas. A gradual increase avoids this problem.

VEGETABLE SLAW

Even people who are not health conscious like this vegctable slaw, which is sweet, crunchy, and beautiful to look at. It is the dish I invariably take to potluck dinners and picnics since it takes ten minutes to make with a food processor and is an impressive-looking dish. If you make too much to eat at one sitting, it will keep four or five days in a tightly closed container. Add the dressing just before serving to keep the vegetables fresh and crisp.

Grate in food processor or with hand grater:

1 raw beet

2 to 3 carrots

¼ to ½ head red cabbage

Mix and serve with an oil and vinegar or Italian dressing.
Makes approximately 1½ quarts.

HUMMUS

(Garbanzo Bean Dip)

I have adapted this traditional Middle Eastern dip to the Anti-illness Diet by reducing its fat content considerably. Usually made with a lot of olive oil, the taste of this hummus recipe does not suffer at all by omitting the oil completely. If you want a little oil in it, use a small amount of cold-pressed safflower. It takes only a few minutes to make this recipe in a blender or food processor and can be served as a dip with crackers or raw vegetables. You can also use it for a sandwich spread. When hummus is eaten with whole grains (bread, crackers, or tabbouli) it becomes a complete protein.

Blend together until creamy:

2 cups cooked (or 1 can rinsed) garbanzo beans

2 cloves garlic

2 tablespoons tahini (sesame butter, found in health food stores and some delicatessens)

juice of ½ lemon

Makes 2 cups.

TABBOULI
(Cold Cracked Wheat Salad)

Tabbouli is another Middle Eastern dish that keeps well and is quick to make. You can use cracked wheat or bulgur wheat, but don't use couscous, which is bulgur (or whole wheat) stripped of its nutrients. Because the wheat has been cracked and pre-cooked, tabbouli requires no additional cooking.

Soak 2 cups cracked wheat or bulgur in 1 cup warm water for 1 hour.
Mix with:

2 chopped tomatoes

½ cup chopped onion or scallion

1 cup chopped parsley

1 cup (or less) lemon juice

½ cup cold-pressed safflower oil

Makes 4 cups.

PASTA PRIMAVERA
(Cold Pasta Salad)

By combining whole grain pasta, lightly steamed vegetables, and a dressing made with cold-pressed safflower oil, you make a healthy and satisfying dish. Use it as a starting point and create interesting variations by adding artichoke hearts, black olives, and chunks of chicken or white meat tuna packed in water for an elegant main course. The pasta and vegetables can be cooked in advance, refrigerated, and mixed before serving.

½ pound whole grain pasta

(rice and soy, whole wheat, buckwheat and wheat, or other), lightly cooked

Add:

2 cups lightly steamed vegetables cut in ½-inch pieces (carrots, mushrooms, cauliflower, broccoli, crookneck squash, green or red bell pepper)

Mix with:

½ cup parsley

1 scallion, finely chopped

fresh garlic to taste

Dress with Italian, oil and vinegar, or oil and lemon juice (using cold-pressed safflower oil) dressing.
Serves four to six.

SPICY CHINESE VEGETABLES AND SOBA NOODLES

This is the recipe I created after getting tired of sautéed vegetables and rice. If you like spicy Oriental food, you'll love it. In addition to being delicious served hot, it makes an excellent cold pasta salad. Soba noodles (buckwheat) can now be found in many health food stores. If you live near an Oriental market, you can find them there as well. If you can't find soba, substitute another whole grain pasta.

½ pound soba or whole grain pasta, lightly cooked

2 to 4 cups vegetables, lightly sautéed in a little vegetable oil. The following are particularly good in this recipe: onions or scallions, mushrooms, broccoli, bean sprouts, chinese snow peas, cabbage, chinese cabbage, bok choy, water chestnuts, zucchini.

Mix together:

2 tablespoons Chinese hoisin sauce (contains a little sugar)

1 tablespoon Chinese chili sauce (no sugar added) or other hot sauce

1 tablespoon tamari sauce

Toss noodles, sautéed vegetables, and sauce together.
Serves four.

CHICKEN BREASTS IN WINE AND TAMARI SAUCE

For a hot entrée or cold lunch, this recipe proves that chicken without the skin does not have to be dry and tasteless. White wine and tamari sauce provide both flavor and moisture. The alcohol in the wine is cooked out during the baking, leaving only the flavor. Tamari is a natural soy sauce made without sugar or preservatives. Many commercial brands are unsuitable because of these additives. Because it is salty, I add ⅓ water to my bottle of tamari. Here, you will dilute it in the pan. You can add fresh garlic, onions, carrots, potatoes, and other vegetables before baking for a one-dish meal.

4 chicken breasts, skinned and placed breast down in pan.

Add:

4 tablespoons dry white wine

3 tablespoons tamari sauce

1 tablespoon water

Cover and bake 1 hour at 350.
Serves four.

POPCORN SUPREME

Popcorn doesn't have to be dry and tasteless either. You can add a little butter as long as it's Better Butter. A dear friend who introduced me to the joy of brewer's yeast on my favorite snack has my deep thanks, as does the patient who suggested adding lemon juice for a distinctive kick. The roughage in popcorn makes it an excellent snack. This is only one of many variations for low-fat, salt-free toppings you can use.

4 cups popped popcorn

Mix:

>   **1 tablespoon melted Better Butter**
>   **½ teaspoon lemon juice**

Sprinkle over popcorn and toss with brewer's yeast powder to taste.
Makes 4 cups.

FOODS TO AVOID

The average American will die of heart disease or cancer. The average woman will get osteoporosis. The average premenopausal woman has premenstrual syndrome. Do you want to be healthy or do you want to be average?

We've been hearing for years about foods that are bad for us. We're still eating them, and often in excessive amounts. Although you may have heard some of the arguments that follow, I find it necessary to reiterate them along with some of the more recent medical evidence as it pertains to women's health. In this way, you will have a more complete picture and a better understanding of why you must make some changes in what and how you eat if you want to be healthier.

FATS

Our fat consumption has increased by 30 percent over the last sixty-five years and so have our fat-related illnesses. Studies from forty countries over the past forty years have shown a correlation between a high-fat diet and cancer of the breast, colon, ovary, uterus, and pancreas. In a recent publication, *Progress in Cancer Research and Therapy,* high *total* fat—not just saturated fat—correlated with cancer in women. With the explanation of EFAs comes an understanding that we need *some* unsaturated fats to help regulate cell function, and in the Premenstrual Syndrome Diet in Chapter 5, we find they help eliminate menstrual cramps and other symptoms. Still, the message is clear: your diet should be low in the total amount of fat you eat. We can and must reduce our intake by eating more chicken and turkey (without the skin), more fish, less red meat, less fried food, and fewer dairy products. And we need to include polyunsaturated vegetable oils each day.

There are three basic kinds of fats: saturated, mono-unsaturated, and polyunsaturated. Saturated fats are found in all animal products, including dairy, and two kinds of vegetable oils—coconut and palm kernel. You may not be aware of coconut or palm kernel oils, but you will notice them when you begin to read labels. They are commonly used in baked goods, cereals, crackers, and other processed foods because they are cheaper than unsaturated oils. Saturated fats should be kept to a minimum in your diet.

Mono-unsaturated fats contain some saturated and some unsaturated fats. They are found in olive oil, peanut oil, and some margarines and vegetable shortenings. Of these, olive oil, containing some EFAs, is best. Use small quantities occasionally and concentrate on other vegetable oils for cooking and salad dressing except when you want the flavor of olive oil.

As we've discussed in the description of the Anti-illness Diet earlier in this chapter, the best oils—high in EFAs—are polyunsaturated and include safflower, corn, sesame, soy, sunflower, and most fish oils. Safflower is highest in EFAs and is the one I recommend you use. When it is used in cooking, the heat destroys its EFAs. However, it is still better to use polyunsaturated than either of the other two varieties of oils.

Unsaturated fats are sometimes made saturated through hydrogenation, a process of heating the oil, putting it under pressure, and forcing little hydrogen bubbles into it. The unsaturated oils become saturated with hydrogen and get hard, as is the case in margarine, shortening, imitation milk, coffee whiteners, and peanut butter. This heating process destroys its vitamins, minerals, and EFAs. It also means that margarines and other hydrogenated substances are no better for you than saturated fats, which are known to contribute to disease.

SUGAR

According to Dr. E. Cheraskin, author of books on nutrition and more than 300 scientific papers, high sugar consumption correlates directly with arteriosclerosis and coronary heart disease, gout, diabetes, hypoglycemia, dental caries, periodontal (gum) disease, kidney stones, urinary infection, intestinal cancer, diverticulosis, indigestion, hormone disorders, obesity, and hypertension. A recent survey gathered from twenty-one countries indicates a strong correlation between sugar and breast cancer mortality for women between the ages of forty-five and seventy-four. It does not include those women with breast cancer who survived the disease. The connection between the two seems to be insulin, which is needed in the production of normal breast tissue and is increased with high sugar intake, according to Dr. S. Seely from the University of Manchester Medical School. With added insulin, breast tissue cells can multiply more rapidly.

To be able to digest sugar your body uses thiamine, riboflavin, niacin, piridoxine, pantothenic acid, phosphorus, and magnesium. Since sugar contains none of these, eating it depletes your body. Many people eat foods high in sugar instead of more nutritious foods that contain the vitamins, minerals, and amino acids their bodies need, and the problems are compounded.

Some people have less tolerance to sugar than others. Dr. Sheldon Reiser, chief of the carbohydrate laboratory at the USDA's Human Nutrition Institute, has found that people with a sensitivity to sugar tend to have high cholesterol and triglycerides when they eat a normal amount of sucrose in their diets. Triglycerides are fatty acids stored in the fat tissues that can be made from sugar. People may have dramatic blood sugar fluctuations after eating just a little sugar or honey. They can suffer from exhaustion or persistent headaches beginning anywhere from fifteen minutes to six hours after eating it. Dr. Reiser recommends we decrease our sugar intake from all foods except fruit by 60 percent and get more of our carbohydrates from grains and starchy vegetables. That's a strong recommendation from a doctor with a conservative government agency!

"Sugar" means sweeteners in all its forms: white, brown, raw, and turbinado, as well as honey, molasses, syrups, sucrose, dextrose, maltose, and all the other "-oses." Pure maple syrup, which is absorbed more slowly, is one of the best choices for a sweetener. Still, your total sugar intake should be low. Since a great deal of sugar in its various forms is hidden in processed foods, if you use them read labels carefully. Choose processed foods low in sugars, make more homemade baked goods in which you can control the amount of sweetener, and develop a taste for less sweet foods. As you eat less, you'll want less. My patients repeatedly tell me that their sugar craving leaves after they stop eating sugar for a while. This may take as short a time as a few days or a week, or it could be as long as six months or more. But once you are free from the lure of sugar you won't want as much of it anymore.

WHITE FLOUR, WHITE RICE

Grains were originally refined to keep for long periods of time without spoiling so large numbers of people could be fed. Now we eat them because we prefer their mild taste and don't have to chew them as thoroughly. Unfortunately, refined grains are missing a lot of nutrients found in whole grains.

When wheat is stripped of its bran and wheat germ, it loses twenty vitamins and minerals. The "enriching" process replaces only four of them, and magnesium, vital to women's health because it helps move calcium into the bones and prevents many premenstrual problems, is not one of those. There's not much left for bugs to eat of these devitalized, storageable "nonfoods," and not much for us, either. Rats and other rodents generally thrive on whole grains, but in one research project where rats were fed only enriched white bread, two-thirds died within three months.

When you eat white bread, not only are you getting fewer vitamins and minerals, you have 87.5 percent less fiber than with whole grain bread. White rice is also low in nutrients and fiber. Fiber unblocks our system by providing bulk to help push waste products through our intestines. Low-fiber diets are associated with chronic constipation, diverticulitis, colon cancer, hemorrhoids, varicose veins, gall bladder disease, and diabetes.

High-fiber foods also give you a satisfying feeling of fullness, which means you're less likely to overeat. Instead of adding a tablespoon or two of bran to a glass of water or juice to control constipation or for weight loss, eat whole grain bread, brown rice, millet, or buckwheat with vegetables, along with oatmeal and other whole grain breakfast cereals.

CAFFEINE

Caffeine is a drug present in coffee, tea, chocolate, cola drinks, and a few herbs from South America like maté tea and guarana. It has been significantly linked to incidences of bladder cancer in women as well as increased cholesterol and triglycerides levels. There is strong evidence that caffeine increases the growth of uterine tumors and breast cysts. Women with fibrocystic breast disease who eliminate caffeine from their diet often find the cysts disappear and their breasts return to normal. I have even known women with uterine or ovarian fibroid tumors who were able to avoid surgery by changing their diet and eliminating coffee and other stimulating drinks. Their fibroids either stabilized or shrank.

Caffeine has also been associated with reduced fertility, miscarriages, and stillbirths. Because it is a habit-forming drug with no nutritional value and may cause birth defects, pregnant women are better off not drinking it at all. It stimulates the heart, which can lead to heart problems; increases gastric secretions, which can lead to peptic ulcers; stimulates thyroid hormone secretion, which can produce anxiety; and causes the kidneys to work harder because it acts as a diuretic. Often people drink coffee to counteract constipation because it helps all smooth muscles (including your colon) relax. This places a dependency on the bowels for caffeine when the same results can be achieved by increasing your intake of fiber and water.

An article that originally appeared in the *American Journal of Clinical Nutrition* found that drinking coffee or tea, either with a meal or within an hour afterward, inhibits iron absorption from 30 percent to 64 percent. This is of great concern to all women, whose iron needs increase during menstruation and pregnancy and whose need for iron exceeds that of men. If you need all the iron you can get from your food, don't follow an iron-rich meal with a cup of coffee or black tea!

Although many people have the idea that caffeine alleviates tension, it actually *causes* stress. It can be responsible for both high and low blood sugar reactions, and people with hypoglycemia or diabetes should avoid it. Blood sugar imbalances are stressful and often lead to fatigue, and fatigue is one reason many people drink coffee and other caffeinated beverages in the first place. Drinking or eating foods with caffeine gives you a false feeling of energy and well-being. You are really putting your body under more stress and exhausting your adrenal glands by artificially stimulating them to produce adrenalin. In the long run, you are likely to wear yourself down.

A caution about guarana, an herb now being used as an appetite suppressant in some diet plans and added to beverages as an energizer. Although it may be labeled "no caffeine added," guarana contains more caffeine than either coffee or tea, according to one of the most comprehensive books on herbology, *Materia Medica and Pharmacology,* and it is its caffeine that suppresses appetite and gives energy.

One gram of caffeine a day can produce serious side effects. Some people are more sensitive to it and may have reactions from a single cup or less. One cup of coffee, depending on whether or not it is instant, percolated, or drip, can contain from 66 to 146 milligrams. Cola drinks vary from 65 milligrams for a twelve-ounce can of Coca-Cola to 32 milligrams per twelve-ounce can of Diet-Rite. Black tea (which prevents iron absorption to a greater degree than coffee) can have from 28 to 46 milligrams per cup, while cocoa, which we give our children to drink, has 13.

If you are not ready to eliminate caffeine at this time, begin by cutting down. Eventually you can replace it with more healthful drinks, and if you decide to continue using it, remember that less is better.

There is controversy concerning decaffeinated coffee, which may leave in the liver residues of the solvents used in the decaffeination process. Water-processed decaffeinated coffee, also called Swiss processed, uses steam rather than chemicals to get rid of most of the caffeine. It is the preferred coffee to drink if you want the taste of coffee.

SOFT DRINKS

The phosphorus level of many soft drinks increases their harmful effects, especially for women. Phosphorus, sometimes in the form of phosphoric acid, is added to many soft drinks to keep the bubbles from going flat. It pulls calcium out of the bones by upsetting the body's calcium-phosphorus balance, which can lead to osteoporosis. While diet sodas tend to have less phosphorus than nondiet drinks, they still have enough to cause problems. Women who are concerned about getting soft or brittle bones would be wise to cut back sharply on soft drinks or stop drinking them altogether.

In one survey that looked at the phosphorus content of more than twenty soft drinks, those containing the highest amounts included: Tab, Coke, Diet Coke, caffeine-free Coke, and Mr. Pibb. Pepsi Free, Diet Pepsi Free, Like Cola, 7-Up, and Mountain Dew had none. Fortunately, mineral water, even artificially carbonated brands, does not have added phosphorus. The only phosphorus they contain is the amount found naturally in the water. This makes them an excellent alternative to diet and nondiet soft drinks, especially if they are low in sodium.

Besides leaching calcium from the bones, soft drinks with phosphorus neutralize the hydrochloric acid in your stomach. Since our production of hydrochloric acid decreases with age, soft drinks can further reduce your body's production of this important digestant. If you are suffering from digestive complaints and drink a lot of sodas you may be causing your indigestion—like Susan, a patient who insists on drinking two or three diet colas a day. She has done so most of her life. By the time she reached her mid-thirties, her hydrochloric acid level was so low she became gassy and bloated after eating anything. She continues drinking soft drinks and she is still taking hydrochloric acid tablets after meals to help her digest her food.

ALCOHOL

As women have entered the work force, as we have competed successfully in executive positions, as we have become more overworked and dissatisfied in the home, our alcohol consumption has increased. Alcohol contributes to premenstrual syndrome, accelerates the growth of *Candida* that can lead to vaginitis, contributes to blood sugar irregularities, produces fatigue, and adds to stress, which can result in herpes.

Drinking alcohol slows down enzyme production and can result in poor digestion, especially of fats. Like sugar, alcohol uses up nutrients for its metabolism and leaves your body depleted. It robs you of vitamin C, iron, zinc, folic acid and other B vitamins, vitamin A, and potassium. It can slow down the function of your thyroid, which can make it difficult for you to lose weight, lower your blood sugar and cause fatigue, reduce adrenal handling of all kinds of stress, and raise your cholesterol, triglycerides, and blood pressure.

Depending on your sensitivity to alcohol, you may have these reactions even without drinking much. Heavy drinkers often compound their problems by eating poorly and not taking in enough vitamins, minerals, or protein to restore those that are being used up or destroyed. Even a moderate drinker may not be getting enough good nutrition. Eating better is no insurance, however. Research shows even the very best diet won't protect drinkers from harmful liver disease.

Alcohol makes it more difficult for the liver to work properly. And, if your liver isn't working properly, it is more difficult to produce the enzyme that metabolizes alcohol in the liver. According to Dr. H. Alslaben, a pioneer in preventive medicine, and Dr. Wilfred Shute, known for his research on vitamin E, a healthy liver can handle only two or three teaspoons of alcohol an hour and it can take as long as twenty-four hours to eliminate the alcohol and the by-products from just one drink. If you have an occasional drink you may be getting away without doing yourself much harm. If you're a steady drinker and think you're healthy, you're fooling yourself.

This doesn't mean you should never drink. Although alcohol isn't *good* for you, you may be someone who can drink from time to time. In a twenty-year study of more than 5000 people conducted in Framingham, Mass., blood pressure in nondrinkers was higher than in light drinkers. This may lead us to the assumption that a little alcohol is healthier than too much or none at all. It would be interesting to note other lifestyle differences between these groups before jumping to any solid conclusion. The rule I use for whether or not a drink can be handled easily is: if you are relaxed and don't care whether or not you have it, it's probably all right. On the other hand, if you feel you need or deserve a drink, if you are in the habit of drinking every afternoon or evening, or if you're looking for alcohol to calm you down, you have a problem with alcohol—don't drink.

ADDITIVES AND PRESERVATIVES

There is ample literature exploring the detrimental effects of additives and preservatives. However, I would like to mention a few of them at this time. Artificial coloring, flavoring, preservatives, and highly processed foods have been implicated in numerous problems from cancer to allergies and headaches. Specifically, there are a few you will want to avoid: sodium nitrate, sodium nitrite, and monosodium glutamate (MSG).

Sodium nitrite and sodium nitrate are used in many processed meats to keep bacteria from forming and to give a "healthy" pink color. These chemicals combine with others in the body to form nitrosamines, considered to be carcinogenic substances. They are found commonly in bacon, luncheon meats, ham, sausage, corned beef, salami, bologna, liverwurst, most frankfurters, and smoked fish. They are also present in many alcoholic beverages. Your safest approach would be to eliminate or minimize these meats in your diet. They are exceptionally high in fats and salt and generally not good for you. You can also add 5000 to 6000 milligrams of vitamin C to your diet each day, since it has been found to help prevent nitrosamines from forming in the stomach and no toxic level for vitamin C has been found. However, since a high-fat diet is the common denominator for so many health problems, the high fat content of these meats makes them poor foods for women.

Monosodium glutamate is a flavor enhancer developed in Japan from soy beans. It can cause immediate symptoms of a tightness in the chest, headache, a burning in the back of the neck, and thirst—all of which have come to be called the "Chinese restaurant syndrome." Originally used in the Orient to impart a meaty flavor to a low-meat diet, it is used today to keep flavor in overcooked and processed foods, neither of which contribute to our good health. Very small quantities have been shown to produce brain damage in young laboratory animals.

MSG is added for flavor to numerous processed foods, including canned vegetables, soups, and tuna fish; many salad dressings and mayonnaise; crackers, potato chips, and baked goods; candy; baby food; and processed meats such as hot dogs, bacon, and sausage. It is used in the preparation of Chinese, Japanese, and other Oriental dishes, but you can ask that it be left out of your food—often with success—in Oriental restaurants, which are now becoming more aware of the sensitivity many people have to this additive. It is also used in other restaurants where food is kept warm over a period of time, or to "bring out" the flavor of hamburger, steak, and other meat.

To simplify the subject of chemicals: eat the most natural, least chemically treated foods you can find. If you want more specific information on particular chemicals, The Center for Science in the Public Interest, 1755 S Street, N.W., Washington, D.C., 20009, has an excellent wall chart called "Chemical Cuisine" for $3 that explains which additives are harmful, safe, or to be used with caution.

FOOD SUBSTITUTIONS

Now that you know which foods work best for an Anti-illness Diet, and which ones are to be avoided as much as possible, you can use the following list to make your transition easier. Begin making simple changes: Better Butter instead of margarine or butter, remove the skin from poultry, cut back on sugar and refined grains, and add whole grains. Gradual changes often are more long-lasting than if you revise your entire diet overnight—and the long-lasting changes will make the greatest impact on your health.

FOODS TO AVOID	PREFERRED FOODS
Sweeteners:	**Sweeteners:**
all refined sugars including white, brown, raw, turbinado; artificial sweeteners; honey; corn syrup	small amounts of pure maple syrup; licorice root to sweeten herb teas; small amounts of fruit juice in cereals or baking
Carbohydrates:	**Carbohydrates:**
white flour, "enriched" flour (found in baked goods, bread, crackers, pasta, pizza, cereals); couscous (precooked, hulled cracked wheat); white rice	whole grains including whole wheat (pasta, bread, crackers), brown rice, cornmeal (corn tortillas), oats (oatmeal), rye, buckwheat, millet, triticale; starchy vegetables including potatoes, sweet potatoes, yams, winter squashes, corn
Vegetables:	**Vegetables:**
canned, frozen, deep-fried	raw, steamed, stir-fried in a little vegetable oil
Fruit:	**Fruit:**
canned, frozen, sugared fruit juices and fruit drinks	fresh or baked (apples); unsweetened applesauce; unsweetened fruit jams; small amounts of dried fruit (one or two pieces)

Protein:

luncheon meats (salami, pastrami, bologna, liverwurst, corned beef, and so on); all pork (bacon, ham, sausage); commercial hot dogs; smoked meat and fish; shellfish (shrimp, lobster, crab, and so on)

Protein:

fresh fish, chicken, turkey, Cornish game hens (skin removed); tofu (soy bean curd); small amounts of eggs, veal, and lean beef and lamb; combined plant proteins (rice and beans, whole grain cereal and soy milk, and so on)

Nuts and Seeds:

roasted and salted, smoked, or dry-roasted nuts, seeds, and nut butters; all peanut products

✳Nuts and Seeds:✳

raw unsalted nuts, seeds, and nut butters (except peanut butter); tahini (sesame seed butter)

Fats and Oils:

fatty meats; poultry skin; saturated oils (palm kernel and coconut); margarine; shortening; lard; chocolate; deep-fried foods (including potato chips)

Fats and Oils:

cold-pressed unsaturated oils, especially safflower; Better Butter; avocado; small amount of butter; nut butters

Beverages:

caffeinated drinks (coffee, black tea, maté tea, colas, cocoa); soft drinks with phosphorus added; sugared fruit drinks, undiluted fruit juice; alcohol

Beverages:

herb teas; coffee substitutes (Postum, Caffix, Pero, Pioneer, and so on); a little water-processed decaffeinated coffee; diluted fruit and vegetable juices; mineral water; lots of pure water

Seasonings:

monosodium glutamate; salt; commercial soy sauce

Seasonings:

tamari sauce; herbs; and spices

HOW TO SURVIVE EATING OUT

Once you begin to eat the anti-illness way, you'll face your supreme test when you eat out. No matter where, you will be up against peer pressure, availability of nutritious foods, and your cravings and willpower. It may not be easy at first, but it's possible. Every small victory is a success; every failure is an opportunity to look at the choices that existed and why you made the ones you did. Keep practicing until eating out is easy. Often you will have to compromise. When you find yourself faced with very little choice, be aware of which foods are better than others.

The first rule of survival is: don't go out to eat hungry. Have a small snack before you leave home or eat a few whole grain crackers, raw almonds, or a piece of fruit. Then if your meal or the friends you're meeting are late, you won't have to fill up on bread or rolls and butter. And you won't have to choose the foods that will make you feel better most quickly—refined carbohydrates.

The second rule of survival is: ask for what you want, even if it's not on the menu or on the table. Ask for foods with sauces and dressings on the side. Have the cheese left off a dish. If you're out with friends who insist on having pizza and beer, order a salad, avoid sausage, pepperoni, and other fatty meats, and eat less than you would ordinarily.

A well-known Los Angeles restaurateur expressed surprise to me about the way some of his customers ordered. "I serve men and women who make important decisions in their businesses and don't hesitate to ask for what they want in other aspects of their lives. Yet when they're here they don't ask if we can prepare their food a little differently. The worst that can happen is that we can't do it."

When you eat at a friend's house, find out the menu ahead of time and bring something you can eat rather than a bottle of wine or a box of candy, such as whole grain rolls or dessert made without sugar. (My hallmark is the vegetable slaw that appears in the recipe section of this chapter.) If this doesn't seem appropriate, you can always eat a snack before you go. If anyone notices you're not eating much, explain you ate late that day. Sample all the foods you want and eat small portions of those that fit into your dietary plan.

If you find something irresistible, eat it and pay attention to how you feel later. Keep your portion as small as possible. Remember, you can eat anything if most of your food is good quality, wholesome, unprocessed, and low in fat. If you eat something you know is not good for you, you did not blow your whole diet. You just went off it for the moment. Go back to it as soon as you can. Don't live with a feeling of guilt. Recognize what you did and be gentle with yourself.

After you feel comfortable with the Anti-illness Diet, or if your health concerns won't wait, you can integrate one or more of the modification diets into it. The specific modifications for a variety of women's health problems, from the Arthritis Diet to the Stressful Living Diet, are found in the following chapter.

CHAPTER FIVE

VARIATIONS ON A THEME

Leave your drugs in the chemist's pot
if you can heal the patient with food!
—HIPPOCRATES

T he basic Anti-illness Diet provides a solid foundation for good health; however, when health problems or nutritional deficiencies already exist, your body may need additional help to heal itself. Using specific foods and nutritional supplements can often speed the healing process by creating balance, and balance is health. The key is to know which foods and supplements you are likely to need. This chapter contains nearly thirty separate diets for specific health problems.

There is a temptation to want to do everything at once and combine too many diets with the Anti-illness Diet in an attempt to get better quickly. This can seriously limit the choice of foods you eat and be very frustrating. In some cases, one diet will tell you to emphasize a food that should be avoided in another. Potatoes are an excellent source of carbohydrates for the Strenuous Exerciser's Diet, but turn into sugar too quickly for someone on the Blood Sugar Diet. Work one program thoroughly until you have obtained the results you're looking for, then move on to the next one. The order in which I work with my patients is:

1. The Anti-illness Diet
2. The Good Digestion Diet
3. The diet for whichever health problem is of most immediate concern

My rationale is that you need a good foundation on which to build. The Anti-illness Diet eliminates many of the foods that cause health problems—sugar, caffeine, large quantities of animal fats—and is filled with those that help your body rebuild itself: whole grains, legumes, and fresh vegetables. The next step is to make sure you can digest the foods you eat. If you have any indications in the questionnaires that you have a digestion problem, incorporate the Good Digestion Diet into the Anti-illness Diet for a few weeks before beginning the diet for your greatest health problem.

If you have an immediate concern such as PMS, low blood sugar, *Candida albicans*, or herpes, start by incorporating into your program one principle from the appropriate diet. With PMS, you may decide to reduce or eliminate dairy products, sugar, or animal fats. If you have *Candida*, you can eliminate foods that contain yeast and sugar. Although these changes may not be enough to solve your health problems completely, they will give you a good beginning.

The object of this book is to provide you with information that you can use over a period of time to methodically strengthen all areas in your body. Be patient, and choose one or two diets that fit in easily with the Anti-illness Diet and still provide you with enough foods to select from to ensure success.

Each diet is designed to fit into the Anti-illness Diet. After an explanation of the condition and why the given dietary recommendations are likely to work, specific suggestions appear in three categories: foods to eliminate because they are detrimental to the condition; foods to reduce because they add little to your health; and foods to emphasize because they add the nutrients your body needs to overcome or prevent the problem. Occasionally, one of these categories will be blank. This simply means that no additional information other than the Anti-illness Diet is pertinent or available at this time for the described condition. Some diets diverge from this format—the ABCs of Eating and the Candida Albicans Diet, for example—while other formats lend themselves better to the information.

When you're healthy, you may be able to get the nutrients you need from your food. When you're not healthy or when you are actively seeking to prevent conditions from occurring, supplements can work faster than food alone to bring your body into balance. Nutritional supplements are just that—they supplement your diet. They are not "instead ofs." They cannot replace eating good food. Taking supplements and eating poorly will not make you healthy. A good diet and the right supplementation are, in my opinion, an unbeatable combination. They are the combination I have been using with my patients successfully for years.

Each diet in this section lists vitamin and mineral supplements that have been found to be helpful for particular conditions. Biochemical individuality prevents the doses listed from being accurate for everyone. But the doses do indicate important guidelines based on sound medical research and my clinical experience. When possible, it is always best to discuss the advisability of nutritional supplements with a health-care professional who is familiar with this course of treatment and who can evaluate your condition thoroughly. If you cannot do this, begin with the lowest recommended dosage for several months. If you feel you are not getting the results you are looking for, increase the dosage gradually. Whenever a supplement is mentioned in the following diets, the dosage is once a day unless otherwise indicated.

When particular kinds of supplements (dry versus oil-based vitamins) or specific brands have been found more effective than others, based on laboratory research or clinical experience, they are named. In my practice, I have found some vitamins and minerals that either are not easily absorbed or are of a low quality. When these supplements are taken, no positive changes appear in laboratory tests or in symptoms. When supplements of a higher quality or greater absorbability are taken, a noticeable change can be seen both in patients' health and laboratory tests.

All supplements are not equal in quality, no matter what you have been told. The biochemists and heads of supplement companies I have spoken with have confirmed my own findings. Many of the vitamins and minerals in drug stores, supermarkets, and even health food stores are either low quality or do not break down effectively and are not absorbed well into the body. I have seen indications of a vitamin C deficiency in a young nonsmoker with good eating habits who took 10,000 milligrams of bargain-brand vitamin C a day. When she switched to a different brand, lower doses eliminated her deficiency.

Some supplement companies put fewer vitamins in their tablets than what is shown on the label. I know of one company that has analyzed some of its competitor's products only to find that some ingredients listed on the label were not in the product. Unfortunately, this does not appear to be unusual. One scientist in the industry estimates as much as 75 percent of the supplements sold to the public may either not contain the full amount of the ingredients shown on their labels or have listed ingredients missing from the products. The better-quality supplements I have found are sold directly to health-care practitioners who monitor their patients' progress and adjust dosages as needed. These are the ones I use in my practice. There are some fine products available in stores, and when I have personal knowledge of them, I will give you their brand names. It has not been easy for the public to differentiate high-quality supplements from those of a lower quality, but all this is changing right now.

Dr. Jeffrey Bland, director of the Laboratory for Nutritional Supplement Analysis at the Linus Pauling Institute of Science and Medicine in Palo Alto, Calif., is working on an independent laboratory analysis to provide a similar type of quality control on supplements as the FDA does with drugs and the USDA with food. This laboratory was chosen by the National Nutritional Foods Association (NNFA) and a smaller group of supplement manufacturers, the Council for Responsible Nutrition (CRN), to grant a seal of quality to those supplements that demonstrate excellence, potency, and purity by passing stringent testing. The Linus Pauling Seal of Quality is one way you can recognize an excellent product that contains what the label says and that breaks down well and is easily absorbed in the body. Always choose a supplement with this seal above one that does not have it when you have a choice between several brands.

SPECIFIC SUPPLEMENTS MENTIONED IN THE DIETS

Vitamin C. When additional vitamin C is needed, use the whole vitamin, rather than ascorbic acid alone. Taking ascorbic acid is like drinking strained orange juice. Bioflavinoids, in the pulp and just under the skin of citrus fruit, help the absorption of vitamin C and make capillaries strong, preventing easy bruising. An article in the *International Clinical Nutrition Review* cited research that shows natural vitamin C with bioflavinoids is not only more easily absorbed, it stays in the body longer than synthetic ascorbic acid.

If a patient is coming down with a cold, herpes, or other infection, or if there is any reason to believe there is poor digestion and absorption, I use powdered C rather than tablets. Whenever you take large quantities of vitamin C (more than 4000 milligrams), use one that is buffered with minerals to reduce stomach irritation and loose bowels. Of all the available powdered and buffered vitamin Cs on the market, I have found two that dissolve quickly and easily, making a tasty, effervescent drink: Emergen-C (Alacer) and Lyte-C (Integrated Health). Both are available in health food stores, and both brands produce vitamin C tablets with bioflavinoids.

Vitamin E. Along with some gynecologists, I am concerned about women who take high doses of oil-based vitamin E capsules for the elimination of breast cysts. Because all oils can become rancid, I prefer using vitamin E in a dry succinate form. Dry E made from wheat germ can also become rancid. In addition to possible rancidity, research by Dr. Jeffrey Bland on the absorption of various types of vitamin E indicates the water-soluble dry E is more easily assimilated than the oil based. The results I have obtained with vitamin E have been with the dry form (Tyson & Associates and Seroyal Brands), available only to health practitioners. A similar product of excellent quality is Amino Opti-E (Integrated Health), sold in health food stores. If you cannot find it, choose another dry E succinate.

Essential Fatty Acids (EFAs). EFAs, explained in the Premenstrual Syndrome Diet (under PMT-C), are found in cold-pressed vegetable oils, especially safflower, oil of evening primrose, and some essential fatty acid formulas (capsule and liquid) found in health food stores. Efamol is the brand of evening primrose oil capsules that Dr. David Horrobin used in his research and is of the highest quality. If you decide to use capsules in addition to, or instead of, adding oil to your food, I suggest you use that brand whenever it is available. Efamol capsules are found in pharmacies and health food stores.

Multi-Vitamin/Minerals. The quality of supplements used to balance the deficiencies of PMS is particularly important. PMS formulas have appeared in pharmacies and health food stores, and reports from gynecologists and patients have indicated all are not as alike as their labels. Some result in side effects such as headaches and nausea. In my own practice, I use Optivite for Women, which contains a full spectrum of vitamins and minerals, with extra B_6 and magnesium. I have found fewer side effects and more consistent results with this formula than with its more than two dozen imitators. Optivite was developed by Dr. Abraham and is manufactured under his strict supervision. It is available in pharmacies or by mail from Health Choice, P.O. Box 2004, Redondo Beach, Calif., 90278.

If you try an Optivite imitator and don't get the results you're looking for, switch to the one with a strong track record before giving up. Whenever a multi-vitamin/mineral is indicated, I am referring to the ratio and potencies of Optivite:

Vitamins:

Liposoluble (fat):

Vitamin A (palmitate, water dispersible)	12,500 iu
Vitamin E (d-alpha tocopherol, succinate)	100 iu
Vitamin D_3 (cholecalciferol)	100 iu

Hydrosoluble (sustained release):

Folic acid	200 mcg
Vitamin B_1 (thiamin)	25 mg
Vitamin B_2 (riboflavin)	25 mg
Niacinamide	25 mg
Vitamin B_6 (pyridoxine HCl)	300 mg
Vitamin B_{12}	62.5 mcg
Biotin	62.5 mcg
Pantothenic acid (d-calcium pantothenate)	25 mg
Choline bitartrate	312.5 mg
Inositol	25 mg
Para-amino benzoic acid (PABA)	25 mg
Vitamin C	1500 mg
Bioflavinoids	250 mg
Rutin	25 mg

Minerals:

Calcium (amino acid chelate)	125 mg
Magnesium (amino acid chelate)	250 mg
Iodine	75 mcg
Iron (amino acid chelate)	15 mg
Copper (amino acid chelate)	0.5 mg
Zinc (amino acid chelate)	25 mg
Manganese (amino acid chelate)	10 mg
Potassium	47.5 mg
Selenium	100 mcg
Chromium	100 mcg

Digestive aids (to help break down the supplement):

Amylase activity	15,000 USP units
Protease activity	15,000 USP units
Lipase activity	1200 USP units
Betaine Acid HCl	100 mg

B-Complex. Some B-complex formulas contain much larger amounts of vitamins than the one I use. When you take too much of a vitamin or mineral, the excess has to be eliminated, causing your body to work harder to separate the usable from the excess. In addition, B vitamins are metabolized in the liver, an organ that often needs support rather than extra work to do. Whenever I speak of a B-complex supplement, I mean one which has ratios similar to the ones I use in my practice:

B-complex (Seroyal Brands):

Folic acid	400 mcg
Vitamin B_1 (thiamine)	110 mg
Vitamin B_2 (riboflavin)	55 mg
Niacinamide	165 mg
Vitamin B_6 (pyridoxine HCl)	55 mg
Vitamin B_{12}	100 mcg
Biotin	300 mcg
Pantothenic acid	110 mg
Choline	80 mg
Inositol	50 mg
Para-aminobenzoic acid (PABA)	25 mg
Betaine HCl	50 mg

Digestive Aids. In my own practice, I find a large percentage of people with digestive problems who need hydrochloric acid, digestive enzymes, or both. I am aware that similar information given by Adelle Davis in the 1960s caused people to rush out and take HCl, sometimes resulting in stomach ulcers. It is extremely important that you take HCl *only* if you need it. Some of the information to determine this need is found in the questionnaires (see chapter 3) and the Good Digestion Diet (page 100). If you have any doubt about your need for digestive support, check with your doctor first. You can often improve your stomach's HCl production simply by chewing your food more thoroughly, eliminating liquids with your meals, and not drinking colas.

HCl stimulates the production of pancreatic enzymes that further help digest food, and your liver supplies other enzymes that break down protein, fats, and other substances. Taking digestive enzymes won't cause ulcers, but if you need HCl, they will not solve your digestive problems, either.

In my practice, I use digestive supplements with HCl and enzymes after taking a thorough health history and examining laboratory tests. Since these particular brands are only available to health practitioners, you may want to find a similar strength in another brand.

Betaine Hydrochloride (Standard Process Laboratories):

(Used temporarily when the stomach does not produce sufficient HCl)

Betaine hydrochloride (HCl)	2 grains
Pepsin	2 grains
Ammonium chloride	½ grain USP

Bromelain-Papain (Seroyal Brands):

(Used temporarily when both HCl and digestive enzymes are needed)

Papain concentrate	125 mg
Bromelain concentrate	80 mg
Pancreatin 4x	35 mg
Betaine HCl	200 mg
Glutamic acid HCl	100 mg

Glandular Therapy. Glandular therapy is the use of raw glands and organs of healthy animals in tablet form to help rebuild damaged tissues in the same organs and glands in our bodies. This type of supplementation has been in existence for many years; however, as with other less conventional therapies, there is some controversy surrounding its use. There are doctors who claim that because they contain the whole gland they can upset our hormonal balance. The description of these products from manufacturers indicates any hormones are removed in the drying process. In addition, laboratory tests before and after their use do not disclose any hormonal fluctuations in my patients who used glandular therapy, and I have found them to be very effective in rebuilding weakened areas quickly. In *The Journal of the Nutritional Academy of Nutritional Consultants*, Alan H. Nittler, M.D., reports evidence that ingested glandulars do, indeed, find their way to specific tissues and glands in the bodies of laboratory animals.

The glandulars I use are only available to health professionals, but there are a number of companies that supply others to health food stores. NF Factor is one I have found to be reputable. Of all the available glandulars on the market, you may find adrenal (for stress) and thymus (for the immune system) most valuable. If you do not want to use any of them, you can often get the same results over a period of time with nutrition alone. Glandulars, vitamins, and minerals simply speed up the process.

Amino Acids. All proteins consist of amino acids, but not all amino acids in our foods are available for use if we are unable to digest them completely. We need amino acids to help make hormones, vitamins, and muscle tissues, and at times we are deficient in one or more of them. Like vitamins, amino acids are best taken together, rather than singly, when they can cause other imbalances. Since vitamins and minerals are needed for their utilization, always take a multi-vitamin/mineral when you add amino acids to your program.

Since most of us eat more than enough protein, we do not need to take amino acids unless there is a deficiency, or a need to quickly repair damaged muscle tissues, as may happen in bodybuilding, long-distance running, and other heavy exercise (see the Strenuous Exerciser's Diet). I use them when there is a specific indication.

The best kinds I have found are powdered "free form" amino acids in capsules. Free form means they are already broken down into single molecules and do not need to be digested like meat, fish, eggs, or protein powders. Powder is more easily assimilated than tablets, which must first be dissolved in the stomach. For best absorption, take amino acids on an empty stomach with a full glass of water, half an hour before eating or between meals. Never take them with milk, since dairy products counteract their action.

I look forward to the day when there will be a seal of quality on amino acids. From the response my patients have to some they find in stores, I believe their quality varies greatly. Those I use are of pharmaceutical grade, the very purest, and are distributed to health professionals by Tyson & Associates. A similar quality you can find in health food stores is under the Integrated Health label.

AUXILIARY TREATMENT

When you determine the specific nutrients your body is lacking and provide them in an easily assimilated form, you can get dramatic results. For some people and for some conditions, a change of diet along with vitamins and minerals will produce results that seem miraculous. It will be the answer you have been seeking. For others, it will be an important step in achieving better health.

When different forms of healing—from the self-help techniques of meditation and relaxation exercises to the objective feedback technique of psychotherapy—seem particularly valuable, they are recommended as auxiliary treatment at the end of each diet. When you add one or more to your nutritional program, you enhance the results. In some cases these auxiliary treatments are optional, but at times adding the perspective of a responsible practitioner such as your doctor would be the wisest course to take.

While you may think of your medical doctor as a primary health practitioner, he or she may also be an adjunct to your nutritional program. Some doctors have little knowledge about nutrition, others have a great deal. In both cases, they are excellent people to monitor your progress through laboratory tests and clinical expertise. General practitioners and specialists like gynecologists are valuable additions to your health team. Choose someone who understands your preference for using nutrition as a means of achieving better health, and speak with him or her to determine how you can best work together.

If your doctor is not interested in nutrition, there are other health practitioners who will be more familiar with your approach and who may be very willing to work with you. Their techniques may seem unusual if you have not experienced them, but they are based on systems of healing that have been used successfully for generations. I encourage you to explore them.

Acupuncturists use a system of Oriental medicine that includes nutrition and are familiar with the way specific foods help the body repair itself. They use a variety of methods to move energy to specific areas such as massage, herbs, and placing extremely fine needles in areas where energy is "stuck" and cannot reach the organs or glands in sufficient supply for healing to take place. An acupuncturist can monitor your progress on your nutritional program and assist your body's natural healing ability by helping this energy get where it's needed.

Some doctors and dentists use acupuncture for pain control, but it is a complete system of healing that goes far beyond this one area. If you are interested in having an acupuncturist work with you but are wary of needles, speak with him or her about your concern. I have often found acupuncture to be painless, and when it is a little uncomfortable the discomfort is greatly outweighed by the calmness, energy, and results I feel after a treatment.

Many chiropractors have studied nutrition in depth in school, and for some it is an integral part of their treatment. They are likely to be familiar with much of your nutritional program and can also monitor your progress. The techniques they use are based on the theory that when the bones in your spine (vertebrae) are in proper alignment, the nerves that pass between them can stimulate each of the organs they go to. The information that nerves send to organs and glands affects their function. If there is pressure or irritation on the nerves that go to the stomach, for example, you may have an overproduction or underproduction of hydrochloric acid. In this case, chiropractic adjustments could help improve your digestion.

Chiropractic can help all of your glands and organs to function better by removing the cause of any pressure or irritation on nerves. Some doctors of chiropractic use slight force to put bones back into place, while others use a more gentle, nonforce techique. Applied kinesiology is one chiropractic technique that specifically incorporates nutrition into its program. Ask a chiropractor which type he or she uses, and choose the one you feel most comfortable with.

If you prefer using medical doctors exclusively, osteopaths are doctors who concentrate on freeing the blood supply to organs and tissues by spinal manipulation. They are trained in adjusting techniques as well as medicine. Some may concentrate more on medicine, while others may focus more on adjusting. Again, talk with the practitioner you are thinking of using to determine their scope of practice and their thoughts on using nutrition to bring balance and health to your body.

Psychotherapy is a large field, encompassing many theories and techniques to help you better understand yourself. Because we tend to abuse our bodies with foods that taste good and deplete us (like sugar, colas, and fats) or overeat to fill ourselves with food when we want to be filled with love, it is often helpful to assist the healing benefits of foods with the objectivity of a trained, licensed therapist. Some therapists do not consider how food affects our emotions, while others are aware of the relationship between the two. If you are pursuing a nutritional approach to better health, it is important to choose a therapist who understands and supports your point of view. The specific methods he or she uses may be less important than their ability to understand you and help you see how your emotions have contributed to your physical problems.

As you begin to develop new eating habits, you may find you are less comfortable around friends who do not think about the foods they eat, or you may feel angry and deprived with the choices that remain. A therapist can help your transition into new patterns, allowing you to focus on the freedom that comes with good health. Don't hesitate to work on your emotional problems at the same time you're concentrating on the physical ones. There is often a psychological reason for eating your way into a health problem, and psychotherapy may be just the nutrition you need for your emotions.

Biofeedback is a technique that teaches you how to be aware of stress inside your body by hearing or seeing how your heart rate or skin temperature changes before, during, and after relaxation using an electronic monitoring device. Once you are aware of how stress affects your body, and you can recognize its subtle signals, you can relax without hearing or seeing feedback from the biofeedback machine. A person trained in biofeedback knows many relaxation techniques and can help you in this interesting and beneficial process.

The benefits of using meditation and relaxation techniques to enhance other forms of healing have been thoroughly explored. There is no doubt that they are valuable adjuncts to any health-care program. Two of the pioneers in this field are Carl and Stephanie Simonton, who began working with terminal cancer patients, using visualization techniques to help them heal themselves. Their success was high enough to impress many in the medical community, and their work can be utilized for people with less serious illnesses as well. For more information, read *Getting Well Again,* by Carl Simonton, M.D., Stephanie Matthews-Simonton, and James Creighton.

One of the most simple books I've seen on how to meditate is *Om, A Guide to Meditation and Inner Tranquility*, by Frank MacHovec. This slim volume, published by Peter Pauper Press, takes only a few minutes to read. You can begin tapping some of the peaceful places inside you immediately using the information it contains.

If you are one of many people who would rather be taken by the hand and led into meditation or relaxation, your solution could be *Mastering Stress,* a cassette tape that teaches "the gentle art of relaxation" on one side and takes you on a "journey to your private paradise" on the other. This is a lovely tape designed by professional health practitioners, available for $11.50 (including postage) from On Course, Inc., 2223 Main St., Suite 49, Huntington Beach, CA 92648.

Of all types of exercise, yoga is one of the most rewarding. Hatha yoga strengthens your body using isometrics, a method of isolating and tensing specific muscles, breathing techniques, and body awareness; as one yoga teacher says, "Hatha [physical] yoga is the first rung on the ladder. It puts your body house in order. After hatha, you can go on to other forms of yoga that interest you." The breathing of yoga helps you focus and release tension as well as balance your body and mind. Look for a yoga teacher who knows anatomy and with whom you have a rapport, and who teaches in a well-ventilated room. Yoga can be an excellent foundation for runners, swimmers, and women engaged in other sports activities. Add it to aerobics exercise for a complete physical workout program.

Exercise is essential for a healthy body. Do whatever exercise you can. Walking or riding a stationary bike fit most lifestyles and health conditions. There is always something you can do to tone sagging muscles and to develop strength in weak areas. If you have physical limitations, speak with your doctor before beginning any exercise program, and always start slowly. Personal experience taught me that too much exercise too soon serves no purpose and only results in the pain of pulled muscles. An excellent book to help you begin exercising is *The Sports Doctor's Fitness Book for Women* by John L. Marshall, M.D., a doctor of sports medicine. It is well illustrated, easy to read, and contains a section for women over forty-five that provides an effective program designed to give noticeable results safely.

You now have sufficient information to incorporate the following diets into the Anti-illness Diet. It's time to get down to specifics.

DIETS FOR CHRONIC CONDITIONS

THE RECOVERING ALCOHOLIC'S DIET

There is no diet for the alcoholic who is still drinking, because medical research indicates that a good diet alone will not prevent liver disease or nutritional deficiencies while abusive drinking continues. As long as you are an active alcoholic, some vitamins are being used to break down alcohol in the liver, others are not being metabolized properly, and some vitamins and minerals are being eliminated too quickly. For this reason, recovering alcoholics are often malnourished and unable to handle the foods their bodies need for repair.

In small quantities, alcohol is a fuel; in larger amounts, it is a poison that deprives the brain of nutrients, destroys brain cells, and robs you of vitamins and minerals. Alcohol is a form of sugar that is absorbed directly into the bloodstream, affecting your central nervous system and blood sugar levels. When you consume large amounts of sugar, your pancreas is called upon to produce insulin to eliminate some of it. The liver is expected to store some for the future, when it is needed.

But alcohol is toxic to both the liver and pancreas, which consequently often don't function properly in alcoholics. Sudden fluctuations in blood sugar levels can produce either hypoglycemia (low blood sugar) or hyperglycemia (diabetes). Many doctors believe all alcoholics are hypoglycemic, even before they begin drinking, and that a genetic inability to use sugar often leads to alcoholism. As a recovering alcoholic it is important for you to realize you may have a blood sugar imbalance. While this diet is designed for the recovering alcoholic who may be hypoglycemic, you may also want to refer to the Blood Sugar Diet for more information.

In addition to storing sugar, your liver uses zinc and some B vitamins to break alcohol down into chemicals your body can use, but it can only do this easily at the rate of one drink an hour. If you keep on drinking, your liver may eventually become fatty and have difficulty metabolizing alcohol. Some liver cells also die and are replaced with scar tissue. This process of slowly destroying the liver is called cirrhosis.

Alcohol so severely impairs the digestion and absorption of nutrients that even the rare alcoholic who eats well is left nutritionally depleted. Good nutrition alone will not prevent serious nutritional deficiencies, because alcohol slows down the production of pancreatic enzymes, which help digest proteins, fats, and carbohydrates. Alcohol also reduces the permeability of our small intestines, which means we do not absorb as many vitamins and minerals as we may think, particularly vitamin B_{12} (needed to help utilize iron), thiamine (needed for a healthy nervous system), and folic acid. A lack of folic acid can produce anemia, common in alcoholics, because alcohol interferes with folic acid metabolism in the bone marrow where red blood cells are made. Folic acid is also used by liver tissues to repair themselves. Naturally present in dark green leafy vegetables, this important vitamin is often missing in the diet of many alcoholics. As a recovering alcoholic, you are possibly deficient in folic acid and need a diet with plenty of vegetables to begin restoring its balance.

Selenium levels are often low. This mineral is found in high-protein foods such as meat and legumes, which are not common in diets of alcoholics. A liver ravaged by alcohol has difficulty digesting and absorbing selenium. It preserves the elasticity of tissues, so when it is depleted, your skin sags and gets wrinkles, aging you prematurely.

While alcohol supresses digestive enzymes, it increases hydrochloric acid in the stomach. This can lead to ulcers and other gastric distress. Fat digestion may be poor, because in addition to a lack of pancreatic enzymes, a damaged liver may produce fewer bile salts, which help in the digestion and utilization of fats. The recovering alcoholic should be on a low-fat diet for at least a year while the liver is repairing.

More consideration is now being given to the connection between alcoholism and genetics. If your parents were alcoholics and you have a drinking problem, there may be a genetic predisposition to alcoholism in your family. Begin to look for this association in your own life and educate your children to this possibility. A genetic inability to regulate blood sugar easily or adrenal gland fatigue may lead to alcoholism.

Alcoholism is a disease of stress. Stress causes the adrenal glands to pump hormones into the bloodstream that suppress the secretion of insulin and release stored sugar in the liver and muscles. This may result in either high or low blood sugar fluctuations that, in turn, cause more stress. Low blood sugar creates a physiological craving for sugars, starches, or alcohol that often cannot be resisted. One amino acid, l-glutamine, effectively eliminates the physiological craving for alcohol and other sugars. Its use has been well documented by Dr. Roger J. Williams, and I have been pleased with the results obtained with my patients who have used this supplement to break their sugar craving. Recovering alcoholics, hypoglycemics, and women with premenstrual sugar cravings have been able to break their sugar habit using l-glutamine.

If you are a recovering alcoholic, your adrenal glands are exhausted from nutritional, chemical, and emotional stress, whether or not you originally had an adrenal gland deficiency. A measurable loss of adrenal gland tissue has been found in autopsies of alcoholics. It is important for you to support these glands with a sound nutritional program and such nutrients as vitamin B complex and zinc, needed for good adrenal function and usually in short supply in alcoholics.

As disheartening as all of this may seem, the damage caused by alcoholism *can* be greatly reduced—and often repaired—with the help of good nutrition and supplementation. Your liver has an incredible ability to rebuild itself, and your body is constantly working to keep itself in balance. With the replacement of depleted nutrients, your body can begin to heal.

Not enough can be said about the need for psychological support in addition to nutritional support. It can be the difference between your drinking and being sober. Both Alcoholics Anonymous (AA) and individual psychological counseling are known to be effective in helping the alcoholic stop drinking. Whether or not you think you need psychological support, you do. If you are serious about remaining sober, seek this out.

One of many successful studies combining nutritional therapy with psychological support, reported in the *International Clinical Nutritional Review*, indicated that 81.3 percent of the people using combined therapies remained sober after six months while only 37.8 percent of those with psychological help alone were sober. In another study of between 20,000 and 25,000 alcoholics, the cure rate was from 50 percent to 80 percent for those on megavitamin therapy. Good nutrition will not only help keep you sober, it will help you become healthy, as in Susan's case.

Susan was a 40-year-old alcoholic who had been drinking for five years, stopping once briefly, then resuming. Her psychiatrist was helping her gradually cut back on her alcohol consumption, but I was concerned that this method would take too long. Her reduced intake still meant she was drinking almost half-a-gallon of wine a day.

A series of blood and urine tests revealed serious nutrient deficiencies, hypoglycemia, high cholesterol, a toxic and fatty liver, and digestive problems. In addition to supplementation, I put Susan on a program to regulate her blood sugar and asked her to eat regularly throughout the day. She was not ready to stop drinking, but she agreed to eat and not increase her drinking.

Eating good food on a regular basis helped, but other factors were contributing to her drinking problem. She discovered drinking alcohol was part of a pleasant ritual she wasn't willing to give up, so she substituted drinking herb tea. With the help of l-glutamine, she lost her physical craving for alcohol, felt better, and looked healthier. But she was still psychologically addicted. Reluctant to go to an AA meeting, Susan agreed to speak with a former patient of mine who was active in the group. The two women had a good rapport, and Susan felt comfortable enough to attend some meetings with her. The combination of better nutrition, supplements to correct deficiencies, changing the content but keeping the ritual she so liked, and AA worked. She has been sober ever since.

It was a victory for Susan to stop drinking, and an equally important one to regain her health. She was not satisfied just to stop drinking. On the Recovering Alcoholic's Diet, she lost weight and felt wonderful.

Why the Recovering Alcoholic's Diet Works: It emphasizes complex carbohydrates, which help regulate your blood sugar, and it reduces fats and proteins, which are hard to digest. The diet eliminates foods that contain sugar or are high in natural sugars, such as fruit juice; they can upset your blood sugar and result in alcohol cravings. It also eliminates foods containing caffeine, preservatives, or other chemicals that nutritionally tax a liver already stressed by alcohol abuse.

Specifics of the Recovering Alcoholic's Diet: Your body has been harmed by alcohol. It needs the best quality foods you can find. This means finding alternatives to fast-food restaurants that use high-fat (pizza, french fries, fried chicken, hamburgers, hot dogs, ice cream), refined (hot dog and hamburger buns, most bread, cakes, doughnuts, cookies), chemicalized foods. You need to eat whole grains (bread, brown rice, pasta) and legumes (lentils, beans, peas) frequently throughout the day. Eat small quantities every four hours (whole grain crackers and bean dip, for example).

Eliminate	Reduce	Emphasize
all alcohol	honey	whole grains
all refined sugars	fruit	legumes
fruit juice	caffeine	fresh vegetables
hot dogs	proteins	herb tea (especially
fried foods	all fats	chamomile)
cheese		popcorn
fatty meats		eating every four hours
potato and corn chips		water throughout the day

If you would like more dietary information, I recommend *Eating Right to Live Sober*, by Katherine Ketcham and L. Ann Mueller, M.D., as an excellent adjunct to the information in this chapter. It is clearly written and contains pertinent, supportive explanations for being on a nutritionally sound diet. One of the best books on the subject is *The Prevention of Alcoholism Through Nutrition*, by Dr. Roger J. Williams. You may want to examine both of these books before deciding which is most pertinent to your case.

Supplements: In addition to dietary changes, to rebuild depleted nutrients and help your body eliminate the fats that have accumulated in your liver, nutritional supplements are important. If you still crave alcohol, use the amino acid l-glutamine to stop that craving and enable you to break your drinking cycle.

I realize I recommend a lot of vitamins and minerals, but most recovering alcoholics have weakened or damaged their body considerably. It may take as long as a year—or longer—of taking these supplements before you can reduce them to a maintenance level of half the given amount.

L-glutamine. Sprinkle 1500 milligrams over ½ piece of fresh fruit two or three times a day. Limit your daily fruit intake to two pieces, eating half a piece at a time. As soon as your desire for sugar or alcohol is gone, stop taking L-glutamine and use only if the craving returns. This amino acid is slightly sweet and combines well with fruit, or take it with herb tea or plain water.

Pancreatic enzymes after each meal to help your body digest proteins and fats.

Multi-vitamin/mineral to replace those washed out of your body by alcohol, missing from your diet, or unable to be absorbed.

Zinc for adrenal gland support; 15 milligrams twice a day (including the amount in your multi-vitamin/mineral).

Brewer's yeast for extra selenium and chromium, used for blood sugar balance. It also contains B vitamins for energy. One-half teaspoon, increased gradually to two tablespoons, a day.

Vitamin C. 1000 milligrams three times a day after meals.

B-complex, 50-milligram formula. Take one twice a day after meals for energy and liver repair. In addition, supplement with the following individual B vitamins to reach the recommended total:

Thiamine (B_1). A total of 2 to 5 milligrams/day.
Riboflavin (B_2). A total of 2 to 5 milligrams/day.
B_6 (pyridoxine). A total of 30 to 50 milligrams/day.
Folic acid, to help prevent or eliminate anemia. 1 to 4 milligrams/day.
Pantothenic acid, to help adrenal exhaustion and depleted supplies. 100 milligrams three times a day for three months; then, fifty milligrams/day total.
Choline, to break down fat in the liver. 500 milligrams three times a day.
Inositol, to work with choline. 500 milligrams three times a day.

Vitamin A. 10,000 iu a day. Your liver may need more than this amount, but additional doses should be administered by a trained health-care practitioner, since high levels are toxic.

Auxiliary Treatment:

Medical doctor or nutritionist: Needed to order and evaluate blood tests that will reveal clinical abnormalities and to monitor your progress. This should be someone who understands your desire to use a nutritional approach and who is familiar with vitamin and mineral therapy.

Psychotherapy: AA or individual counseling is a necessary adjunct to nutritional therapy. It is important to come to terms with any self-destructive patterns and feelings of unworthiness, which are often present in alcoholism, that you may have.

Acupuncture: This can work to help strengthen your liver, usually the organ most damaged by alcohol, to improve your digestion as the enzymes begin to work, and to alleviate symptoms of lethargy and irritability as you continue to improve. Acupuncture can help you relax, sleep better, and give you more energy to support the changes you are going through.

Exercise: This helps tone muscles, moves toxins out of your body more rapidly, and gets your energy flowing. A brisk half-hour walk each day, along with ten minutes of stretching, is sufficient. As you become healthier you can add other, more strenuous exercises.

Massage: Helps eliminate toxins, energizes your body, and helps you get in touch with how you feel. Alcohol cuts off your feelings, and it is important for you to learn to trust, to be open, and to be willing to be vulnerable. Allowing someone to touch you in a loving, nonsexual way can be an important step in feeling worthwhile and opening up to the healing process.

THE FOOD ALLERGY DIET

For purposes of this book, an allergy is probably more accurately described as a food sensitivity or intolerance. It is any adverse reaction to a food that occurs whenever you eat it. A reaction may be caused by such factors as poor digestion, low immunity, or exhausted adrenal glands. When this is the case, you may be successful in identifying the causes for your allergic symptoms, treating them, and becoming allergy free.

I am not an allergist. The information in this section is condensed into a simple approach that I have found works well with many of my patients. It does not contain all you necessarily need to know about allergies. If your condition is more complex and does not respond to the techniques described here, you may want to seek help from a medical doctor or chiropractor—health-care professionals who are familiar with other approaches to solving allergy problems.

William Crook, M.D., allergy specialist and author of *Tracking Down Hidden Food Allergy*, believes you are most likely to be allergic to the foods you eat daily. Many other experts agree with his findings. In my practice, I often ask patients to name the three foods they would not want to be stranded on a desert island without. Those are the first foods we eliminate and are often the cause of their problems.

In a sense, we have more a physiological than a psychological addiction to the foods that cause our allergic reactions. This is how it works. Any type of addiction, from drugs to coffee to food, causes withdrawal from a few hours to three days after ingestion. The withdrawal may be such reactions as depression, irritability, anger, or headaches. As soon as we eat the addictive food our systems disappear and we feel better—until we need another "fix." You may be addicted to something as common as coffee, sugar, wheat . . . or chocolate.

There are several conditions that provoke allergies, according to Alan Levin, M.D., and Merla Zellerbach in *The Type 1/Type 2 Allergy Relief Program*. You may have a fixed allergy, which means you get a reaction whenever you eat a particular food in any quantity. You may have a cumulative allergy and only get symptoms after you eat the food in large quantities. At times, however, even small amounts of allergic substances cause severe reactions. People with yeast allergies can feel terrible after eating salad dressing made with vinegar, which contains small quantities of yeast. Or you may have a variable allergy and never know when you are going to have a reaction because it can be based on a number of other factors. For example, your wheat allergy may not cause you any problem if you eat a piece of bread indoors, but if you eat it outdoors on a day when there is pollen in the air, you might have a reaction. These allergies are particularly difficult to identify. If you want to track down the source of your food sensitivities, be aware of these varying situations. A food allergy can exist even if you don't have symptoms every time you eat a particular food.

In an article on food sensitivity in *Nutrition Reviews*, Dr. Charles D. May believes that 90 percent of food allergies come from milk, eggs, nuts, and wheat. To this, other experts add sugar, corn, soy, caffeine, alcohol, and yeast. Combined, they consist of the most common ingredients in our diet, yet many people live easily without eating one or more of them.

A major cause for food allergies is poor digestion: insufficient or diluted digestive juices (see chapter 1 for a discussion of hydrochloric acid). Gastric juices also trigger the production of enzymes from the pancreas that not only help us digest food, but also control all kinds of inflammation, from cuts and bruises to food allergies. Without enough enzymes you can't digest your food completely or be protected against the inflammation caused by allergic reactions resulting from incomplete digestion.

Incomplete digestion can also be responsible for lowered immunity and tired adrenal glands, also contributors to allergic reactions. The adrenal glands produce hormones that leap to our defense when foreign substances are present in our bloodstream. They may be harmful bacteria or simply partially digested food, perhaps some chicken. These hormones throw a protective shield around the particle, which could otherwise cause irritation and inflammation to delicate tissues. Our white blood cells, the immune system's knights in shining armor, get on their horses, find the captured invaders, and kill them. The undigested chicken is destroyed; our immune system has won another victory. However, if you are allergic to chicken, another battle will begin with your next bite.

When you have allergies there is a war going on inside your body. Your allergic reactions are a response to the battle and the devastation caused when sensitive tissues are damaged. Not only is there a strain on the immune system, constantly called upon to "kill" pieces of chicken, bread, cheese, and other partially digested foods, your adrenal glands become tired from producing so many hormones. If there are too many or too few of them, they will not respond to the irritants, and you will have an allergic reaction.

At 45, Bobbie suspected she had had a dairy allergy for years, but she was never willing to face it and stop eating her favorite food—cheese. Whenever she had dairy products she got bloated and gassy, her nose was stuffed in the morning, and she went to sleep at night with mucous in her throat. After eating meals containing a lot of dairy products, she became so sleepy she had to take a nap. None of this discomfort was enough to get her to stop eating dairy products, but when she was told her premenstrual anxiety and moodiness would go away if only she would stop for a while, she agreed. Bobbie began taking digestive enzymes to help her digestion and a vitamin-mineral formula for PMS, which also supported her adrenal glands.

Three months later her PMS was gone, and she was told she could add small amounts of dairy products back into her diet. But her craving had left. She ate some occasionally, but binged on cheese only once. That episode left her with her familiar symptoms of gas, bloating, a stuffed nose, mucous in her throat, and fatigue. Instead of making dairy products a substantial part of her diet, as she had in the past, Bobbie only eats a little, and not every day. She has found that as long as she keeps the amount low, she has no PMS and no allergic reactions.

Why the Food Allergy Diet Works: It works on three levels. First, it identifies and temporarily eliminates the offending food—whatever is causing your allergic symptoms. Next, it strengthens the digestive system by providing you with digestive enzymes and HCl after meals for a few months, to assure that you are digesting your food. When your digestion is better and there are fewer battles inside your body, you are taking stress off the immune system. Finally, it strengthens your adrenal glands by eliminating the stress of continual hormone production triggered by foods you react to.

Specifics of the Food Allergy Diet: Identify as many foods as possible that give you allergic symptoms by using the health diary and pulse test. The pulse test, originated by Dr. Arthur Coca, and explained in more detail in his book *The Pulse Test,* is another simple method you can use to identify food allergies. In essence, you count your pulse for one minute just before eating, and three times after eating at half-hour intervals. A difference of one or two beats per minute is often significant for detecting an allergy to something you ate. This increase occurs when an allergy causes adrenalin to be released, and additional adrenalin makes your heart beat faster. Become a detective and separate the foods you eat, eating one at a time over a period of a few days, until you find the responsible culprit.

Once you have identified an offending food, avoid it completely for two or three months while you strengthen your digestive system and adrenal glands with supplements. After that time, you may find you can eat it frequently or occasionally with no repercussions. Sometimes simply avoiding a food is not enough. When this is the case, consider the rotation diet with the remaining foods you can eat.

On a rotation diet, you eat a food only once every four days. Foods belonging to the same food group, or food family, can be eaten every other day. The rationale behind this is that you are more likely to become allergic to a food if you eat it frequently, and foods which are chemically similar may produce allergic reactions more easily than those which are less similar. It is not easy to eat out and be social when you are on a rotation diet, or to be spontaneous with food. All meals must be carefully planned and even more carefully prepared. However, it is an excellent way to control allergic reactions while you are strengthening your immune system and adrenal glands. If you would like to try this approach, the following books give details along with lists of foods grouped into food families: *Brain Allergies: The Psycho-Nutrient Connection,* by William H. Philpott, M.D., and Dwight K. Kalita, Ph.D.; *Dr. Mandell's 5-Day Allergy Relief System,* by Dr. Marshall Mandell and Lynne Waller Scanlon; and *How to Control Your Allergies,* by Robert Forman, Ph.D.

Whether or not you go on a rotation diet, it is important to vary your foods as much as possible. Do not eat the same grains, fruit, meat, or vegetables every day. The more variety you have in the foods you eat, the better you will feel once you have eliminated known offender foods. Even if you don't think you have a wheat allergy, for example, use rye crackers one day instead of bread; make wheat-free corn muffins (use all cornmeal instead or part wheat flour) for another day; and buy rice crackers or puffed rice cakes for still another alternative. Vary your cereals to include oats (oatmeal and granola) and corn (corn flakes and grits). Make some salads with a lettuce base, and others with spinach or cabbage. Don't automatically buy the same foods week after week. Look around you to see more choices; read cookbooks to find different recipes. If you usually make chicken, roast a turkey, slice it, and freeze it in small packets for quick non-chicken meals. Bake a yam or sweet potato instead of always using white potatoes.

Choose one or two of your favorite foods and eliminate them from your diet. You will probably experience some withdrawal symptoms for a few days until the substance has completely left your body. Substitute other foods that you enjoy. Life is not as unbearable as you might expect without caffeine, or wheat, or dairy products. When you are free from your food addictions, some or all of your allergic reactions will be gone. Eliminating food allergies can be as complicated as a rotation diet, or as simple as avoiding a food or group of foods.

The following are samples of a few common diets for allergy-free eating:

The Dairy-Free Diet:

Instead of:	Substitute:
using milk on your cereal	soy milk or diluted apple juice
using milk or cream in baking and other cooking	soy milk (powdered is fine for baking, gravies, and other recipes)
drinking milk as a beverage	diluted fruit juice, water, cold mint tea (or other herb tea)
cheese in casseroles	tomato sauce, oil, tamari sauce
ice cream	soy-based frozen desserts, such as Ice Bean and Ice Dream
butter	usually causes no reactions

The Wheat-Free Diet: Wheat flour is both fine and glutinous (sticky), which makes it an excellent grain for baking light baked goods that don't fall apart. On a wheat-free diet you can substitute other grains for wheat, but they must have similar properties for the finished product to look and taste right. Rice flour is very fine but not glutinous, while oat flour (oatmeal ground dry in a blender) is heavier but glutinous. I often combine the two. You can add other flour to a mixture, such as cornmeal, buckwheat, millet, and rye, but be aware that different flours have different properties. Fortunately, there are a number of excellent cookbooks to help you make this or other allergy diets work. I like *The Allergy Self-Help Cookbook*, written by Marjorie Hurt Jones, R.N., as well as *Good Food, Gluten Free*, by Hilda Cherry Hills, written specifically for wheat- and other gluten-free diets. You may also find *The Allergy Cookbook and Food-Buying Guide*, by Pamela P. Nonken and S. Roger Hirsch, M.D., and *Dr. Mandell's Allergy-Free Cookbook*, by Fran Gare Mandell, M.S., valuable additions to your cookbook collection.

Instead of:	Substitute:
shredded wheat and other wheat cereals	wheat-free cereals like Cheerios, oatmeal, some granola, puffed rice and corn, corn flakes, and so on.
bread	wheat-free breads (found in health food stores)
crackers	rice or rye crackers made without wheat, corn tortillas if available
breaded fish or chicken	cornmeal, oat bran, and so on for breading
cakes and cookies	buy wheat-free in health food stores or make your own, using other flours (rice, oat, millet, small amounts of buckwheat or rye)
gravy thickened with wheat	butter and lemon, tomato sauce, or gravy thickened with rice flour

The Yeast-Free Diet: See the Candida Albicans Diet in this chapter.

Supplements: Two levels of supplements can assist you in overcoming your food allergies while you avoid those foods that cause reactions: enzyme therapy and vitamin/mineral supplementation. The enzyme therapy is to assist your body in its production of HCl and pancreatic enzymes (sometimes called proteolytic enzymes). You may only need to use it for two or three months. If you need to take digestive support for a longer time, reduce the amount you take.

Vitamin and mineral supplements can assist your immune system and adrenal glands. B vitamins are among the most important; however, most are made with yeast. If you have allergies, be extra cautious and buy only high-quality, yeast-free vitamins. A multi-vitamin/mineral formula may be sufficient, but I have found higher quantities, taken for two or three months, is especially helpful when allergic reactions have been severe. Most vitamins will state whether or not they contain yeast in them. Optivite does not contain any yeast, and is a safe multi-vitamin/mineral to use on this program. The supplements I use in my practice are supported by William Philpott, M.D., and Dwight Kalita, Ph.D., in their book *Brain Allergies: The Psycho-Nutrient Connection.*

Enzyme Therapy:
After meals—a digestive enzyme tablet containing:
60 to 70 milligrams pancreatin (4x)
160 to 200 milligrams betaine HCl
25 to 45 milligrams pepsin
50 to 75 milligrams papain

Before bed (may be taken on an empty stomach):
300 to 900 milligrams pancreatin without HCl

Vitamin and Mineral Support:
Multi-vitamin/mineral containing at least:
300 milligrams B_6
60 micrograms B_{12}
200 micrograms folic acid
1500 milligrams vitamin C
Trace minerals

For more severe problems, add the following for two to three months:
500 milligrams B_6 three times a day
400 to 800 micrograms folic acid three times a day
250 to 500 micrograms B_{12} three times a day
1000 milligrams vitamin C four to six times a day

Auxiliary Treatment:

Medical doctors: If your allergies are severe and do not respond to the above suggestions, seek medical care. There are many kinds of allergy specialists who use a variety of treatments. One type of doctor, called a clinical ecologist, can help your immune system become stronger by giving specific antigens, substances that help desensitize your body to the foods that give you allergic responses. To locate this type of doctor, write to the Society for Clinical Ecology, 2005 Franklin St., Suite 490, Denver, CO 80205.

Chiropractic: Your stomach may not be producing enough HCl because of a spinal misalignment or a need for your cranials (the bones in your head) to be adjusted. If this is the case, a chiropractor or osteopath who does cranial adjustment as well as spinal manipulation can help correct the underlying reason for your allergies.

THE ARTHRITIS DIET

Arthritis is an ancient disease that can be traced back millions of years to dinosaurs, whose bones show its damaging effects. Today doctors classify a number of different kinds of arthritis, including osteoarthritis and rheumatoid arthritis (inflammation of the joints), which is often associated with childhood rheumatic fever. Protestations from the medical community to the contrary, rheumatoid arthritis has been helped by nutrition. While a change in diet will not *cure* arthritis, it may stabilize and control it, and uncomfortable symptoms such as swelling and pain may be decreased or even eliminated. The Arthritis Diet is concerned primarily with rheumatoid arthritis.

Rheumatoid arthritis is three times as common in women as in men. Its cause is not positively known, but theories attribute the inflammation of the joints to food allergies and poor lubrication of the joints caused by a lack of synovial fluid, the lubricant that enables us to move easily.

When inflammation occurs in and around the joints, cartilage is eventually destroyed and ligaments are weakened. Whenever there is inflammation, we should look to food allergies and a need for pancreatic enzymes (which alleviate inflammation) as possible causes. Foods implicated in arthritis are the nightshade family (tomatoes, white potatoes, eggplant, and garden peppers), dairy products, red meat, wheat, and citrus.

A sensitivity to the nightshade family may be a toxic reaction to a substance called solanine, which inhibits one of the enzymes that helps keep our muscles flexible. Solanine is not destroyed by water or heat. It remains active at all times. Livestock that eat the leaves of plants containing this chemical get calcification in their soft tissues. This may be because the active ingredient of vitamin D, known to contribute to arthritis, is in these plants. The similarity between soft tissue calcification in livestock eating plants high in solanine, and that caused by high levels of vitamin D, has been seen in research experiments and reported in *The Nightshades and Health*, by Norman F. Childers and Gerard M. Russo, a book concerned with arthritis and its relationship to plants in the nightshade family.

A nightshade-free program for arthritis relief was originally developed by Dr. Collin H. Dong, a medical doctor who found relief both for himself and for hundreds of his patients by totally eliminating all nightshades, including tobacco, from the diet. His clinical experience led him to the discovery that the more recent the arthritis, the sooner symptoms would be likely to disappear on the nightshade-elimination diet—often within three months. However, with bone and vertabrae damage, it could take from nine months to a year before obtaining any results. Subsequent research studies that refute Dr. Dong's work have not been of long enough duration to disprove his findings. I have used Dr. Dong's principles with some of my arthritic patients, and have seen inflammation reduced and eliminated, and painful, stiff joints become flexible and free of pain. While it does not work in every case, I suggest you try it for yourself to see whether or not it can bring you relief.

In addition to the nightshade family, I have found other foods that irritate arthritic symptoms: dairy products, wheat, and citrus fruits. Patients who eliminate these foods often find relief from swelling and pain. After symptoms have been reduced to a level of comfort, citrus and wheat can be reintroduced to see if they cause any reactions. The nightshades and dairy products, however, should be permanently eliminated.

Dairy products have two strikes against them: they are high in both calcium and vitamin D. We have spoken before of women's difficulty in assimilating calcium (see the Premenstrual Syndrome Diet for more details). If it is not mobilized into the bones with the help of magnesium, absent in these foods, it may collect in soft tissues and cause calcium deposits. Vitamin D, added to dairy, accelerates calcification. Too much of it from food, or sunshine, is not wise for the arthritic person.

An extremely interesting case written up in the *British Medical Journal* implicates dairy products very strongly in a case of rheumatoid arthritis where there was no detectable food allergy and no typical food allergy reactions. The woman studied loved cheese, and ate as much as a pound of it every day for eighteen years. When she stopped eating all dairy products, her joint pains eased up considerably, but they returned when she had just a little cheese or milk. Allergy tests were negative except when she ate dairy products. Stay away from dairy products, except a little butter. They are too highly suspect for anyone with arthritis to eat. While this single case is not enough to revolutionize the role of nutrition in arthritis care, it bears repeating for those people who may have similar sensitivities to dairy products.

Although eggs are sold in the dairy section of most markets, they are not dairy products—they don't come from cows. Unless you have a reason to avoid them, they may be very beneficial. Eggs are high in sulfur, a mineral found almost exclusively in this food and often low in rheumatoid arthritis patients, who tend not to like, or eat, eggs very much. If this sounds like you, Dr. Carl Pfeiffer, a prominent research psychiatrist and author of numerous books on health, suggests you eat two eggs a day. Another arthritis remedy using sulphur, used throughout Europe, is to soak in hot mineral springs. Both the heat and sulphur in the water may be beneficial for arthritis pain.

A number of nutrients other than sulphur have been found low in people with arthritis: some of the B vitamins including B_6 and niacinamide, vitamins C and E, iron, magnesium, and zinc. Both vitamin E and zinc are important for a strong immune system, which has the ability to counteract inflammation.

In the early 1940s, Dr. William Kaufman, a New England doctor, found niacinamide was effective in restoring movement to stiff joints. Today, both niacin (which produces flushes after taking in large doses) and niacinamide (which does not) are used to increase flexibility and decrease the pain and stiffness of rheumatoid arthritis. Vitamin B_6 has been used to obtain similar results and can be effective within six weeks of the beginning of vitamin therapy.

Vitamin C works on two levels: to help eliminate iron and copper deposits in the joints and to help produce collagen. Collagen is a sticky, gluelike substance that holds our cells together and is an important ingredient in our spinal discs. While many people with rheumatoid arthritis have low blood iron levels, this mineral may collect in the joints and cause pain. In addition, aspirin, taken for pain control, destroys collagen and lowers the white cell count; vitamin C counteracts these actions.

Arthritis may be a result of calcium malabsorption. When this is the case, magnesium supplementation should be considered, since it helps move calcium out of the soft tissues and joints and into the bones. Since both calcium and iron require hydrochloric acid for absorption, your stomach needs to make sufficient HCl. If calcium is being deposited in and around joints, your blood serum calcium may be low. In fact, a study in England in 1981 revealed lower serum calcium in arthritis patients than those free from the disease. With arthritis, it is important to know that the calcium you are eating is being digested and absorbed, not stored in soft tissues or excreted.

The efficacy of arthritis diets in eliminating pain is steeped in controversy. Some say they work, while others claim they have no effect in reducing swelling, controlling pain, or eliminating symptoms. My clinical experience has shown the Arthritis Diet does work in many cases. Instead of entering into the debate, try the diet for six months and find out for yourself what it can do for you. You can get additional information from *Arthritis: Don't Learn to Live with It*, by Carlton Fredericks, Ph.D. Explore every area you can. You don't necessarily have to live with the pain and discomfort from arthritis.

Why the Arthritis Diet Works: It eliminates those foods that have been strongly implicated in causing joint pain, stiffness, and inflammation and at the same time adds foods that supply some of the vitamins and minerals often low in people with this disease. You may want to read the Food Allergy Diet and take appropriate information from it, like using the pulse test to identify food allergies that may be contributing to your arthritic symptoms.

Specifics of the Arthritis Diet: When you eliminate a food or food group like the nightshade family or dairy products, remember that even a small amount of food can cause a reaction. Powdered milk added to frozen dinners, salad dressing with a little tomato, olives with pimiento (red peppers), fish sprinkled with paprika, and most prepared soups, must all be avoided. Potato starch and potato flour should be eliminated as well. Read all ingredients in canned, bottled, and boxed foods thoroughly, and be extremely careful when you eat out. Know the restaurants you eat in, and question the waiter to be certain you are not eating dairy products or nightshade foods hidden in complex recipes. Eat simply and avoid sauces, which may have potato starch as a thickener.

Your arthritis pain and inflammation may respond to a number of dietary changes. Rather than make them all at once, change your diet one stage at a time.

Eliminate	Reduce	Emphasize
Stage I:		
refined sugar	wheat	eggs
white flour	dairy products	whole grains
white potatoes	citrus	fresh vegetables
tomatoes		fresh fruit
eggplant		
garden peppers		
paprika		
tobacco		
Stage II:		
milk	wheat	same
cheese	citrus	
yogurt		
ice cream		
powdered milk		
Stage III:		
wheat	citrus	same
Stage IV:		
citrus		same

Instead of:	Substitute:
white potatoes	sweet potatoes
	yams
	brown rice
	whole grain pasta
	whole grain bread
dairy products	soy milk
	frozen soy desserts
	(nondairy ice cream)
wheat	wheat-free bread and muffins
	rice and rye crackers
	other whole grains
citrus	other fruit
(includes strawberries)	(including other berries)

Supplements: Supplementation is recommended in the following areas: hydrochloric acid (HCl) for better digestion and enzymes for anti-inflammatory action; vitamin E and zinc to help improve the immune system; vitamin C for collagen repair and to chelate unabsorbed iron and copper; specific B vitamins to reduce inflammation and increase flexibility; and a multi-vitamin/mineral that contains good amounts of magnesium, some iron, and the full complement of B vitamins (such as those described at the beginning of this chapter).

Digestion/Anti-Inflammatory:

After meals, take one tablet containing:

60 to 70 milligrams pancreatin (4x)

160 to 200 milligrams betaine HCl

25 to 45 milligrams pepsin

50 to 75 milligrams papain

Improved Immune Response:

400 to 800 iu water-soluable vitamin E

15 to 20 milligrams zinc two times a day

For Arthritis Relief:

multi-vitamin/mineral with twice as much magnesium as calcium, to help mobilize calcium into the bones and out of soft tissues

100 to 500 milligrams niacin after each meal, taken with

1000 milligrams vitamin C, to enhance its effectiveness, plus 1000 milligrams vitamin C every hour until stool becomes loose, then reduce to a level of comfort

50 to 250 milligrams vitamin B_6 for flexibility and pain reduction

Auxiliary Treatment:

Exercise: To help increase circulation and stimulate blood flow. Walking, water exercise (movement in a pool or jacuzzi), and swimming are among the best. It is not necessary to do strenuous exercises, but rather to do something every day to allow blood to circulate throughout your body.

Massage: To increase circulation, decrease stiffness, and relieve pain. If you find it difficult to exercise due to stiffness, you may want to have a massage, or have a friend gently massage your hands or feet, and then do a little stretching. The tensions that come from living with pain can add to your discomfort. Massage is not a luxury for you, it is a necessity.

Acupuncture: To bring increased warmth into hands and feet, to relieve pain, and for increased mobility. Acupuncture can help reduce and sometimes eliminate the pain of arthritis. Even if this pain control is temporary, it can be a relief to be free from it for a while. Continued treatments can bring you more flexibility, increasing your circulation and energy.

THE BLOOD SUGAR DIET: DIABETES AND HYPOGLYCEMIA

Biochemical individuality plays an important role in sugar metabolism. Some people have the ability to handle moderate amounts of sugar with relative ease, while others end up with hypoglycemia or diabetes. A genetic inability to metabolize sugar properly—combined with a diet high in refined sugars, which puts a stress on the blood sugar regulating mechanism—often leads to these two diseases. In the case of diabetes, overweight contributes to it, often resulting from years of eating improperly. A good diet can prevent diabetes even if you are among the one in six people with a biochemical tendency toward diabetes, and a good diet can alleviate and sometimes cure it.

Our blood sugar is regulated primarily by the pancreas, liver, and adrenal glands, which produce hormones that send messages to one another about how to convert the sugar in our foods to energy. Our muscles need sugar for strength, and our brain needs it so we can think clearly. A blood sugar problem, either hypoglycemia or diabetes, means that energy (sugar) is not getting into your cells and providing you with necessary fuel. This is why people with these conditions have symptoms of fatigue, listlessness, and disorientation.

The pancreas is a delicate mechanism with checks and balances to help keep our energy stabilized. It secretes insulin into the bloodstream after we eat. Insulin, by moving sugar from our blood fat and muscle cells and into our liver, where it can be stored until we need it at a later time, lowers our blood sugar. Other chemicals, made by the adrenal glands, raise the sugar in our blood by telling the liver to send it back into our bloodstream when more is needed. When there is a breakdown in any of these areas, our blood sugar may become too low (hypoglycemia) or too high (diabetes). A liver problem, exhausted adrenal glands, or a malfunctioning pancreas can all lead to blood sugar irregularities. It is interesting that an increased amount of atherosclerosis is being found in people with blood sugar handling problems, and people with atherosclerosis are being found to have a higher incidence of diabetes and hypoglycemia. The two seem to go together. By changing your diet, you may be preventing two major illnesses.

Although we are living in a coffee-and-doughnut society, our bodies have not learned how to keep up with our habits. They cannot handle enormous amounts of refined carbohydrates, caffeine, nicotine, and alcohol on a constant basis. These substances overstimulate the pancreas to produce too much insulin, which eventually results in lower blood sugar (hypoglycemia). When the pancreas is too exhausted to respond to the stimulants we take, it gives up and secretes very little insulin, resulting in high blood sugar (diabetes). Although all carbohydrates, including candy, fruit, and rice, stimulate insulin production, the more refined the carbohydrate, the quicker insulin is produced. This is why candy is called a "quick energy" food. It's also fatigue-producing a few hours after it's eaten, however, when the blood sugar is reduced by too much insulin.

Both caffeine and nicotine stimulate the adrenal glands to manufacture hormones that tell the liver to release sugar. The more you drink coffee and smoke cigarettes, the more you deplete your reserve of sugar stored in the liver and put unnecessary amounts into the blood. Excess blood sugar then stimulates your pancreas to make more insulin, and you're caught in a vicious cycle.

A word about marijuana: in my personal and clinical experience, I have not seen any patient who has smoked marijuana on a consistent basis (four or more times a week for six months or longer) who does not have low blood sugar symptoms. Anyone who has smoked it at all is aware of a craving for sugar or starches afterward. Whether or not you give in to this craving, your blood sugar is being altered by this drug. If you have, or suspect you have, any kind of blood sugar irregularity, don't smoke marijuana, even occasionally.

There are two types of hypoglycemia, or low blood sugar—fasting and reactive. Fasting hypoglycemia can come from such sources as liver disease, tumors, and hormonal deficiencies. Often, the best way to solve this problem is to remove the tumor and correct the condition medically. Nutrition plays an important part in this solution, but it may not be the total answer. Reactive hypoglycemia, or having a reaction after eating particular foods, can often be treated with diet alone. It most commonly affects women between the ages of 30 and 40 who have a family history of diabetes, alcoholism, obesity, and mental illness, and it is one of the most common problems I see in women patients.

Approximately 25 million adults in this country suffer from this type of blood sugar imbalance, and many more have less consistent, or less severe, reactions. We will be talking about reactive hypoglycemia, which can come from either a biochemical sensitivity to sugar or from food allergies. While fewer people have clinical hypoglycemia as shown on a glucose tolerance test, I find a great many have drops in blood sugar due to the foods they eat. By correcting their diet, their blood sugar symptoms leave.

There are two types of diabetes—juvenile and adult onset. In both, the pancreas does not produce enough insulin to keep sugar in the bloodstream at the proper level. Too much sugar remains in the blood rather than getting into our cells where it's needed for fuel. The result is fatigue and increased appetite. We will be addressing adult onset diabetes, a disease that responds well to dietary changes. Juvenile diabetes requires taking insulin daily and does not respond to nutrition alone. However, the nutritional information in this chapter pertains to all kinds of diabetes. The adult onset variety may be the result of a genetic weakness, viruses which have damaged the pancreas, obesity (often the result of improper eating habits), stress, or a lack of particular trace minerals such as chromium and zinc. As with hypoglycemia, more women than men suffer from diabetes, and with both, sugar is a contributing factor.

Reactive Hypoglycemia: Symptoms of reactive hypoglycemia are physical and emotional and include feeling tired a few hours after eating, mid-morning and mid-afternoon fatigue, headaches, feeling irritable or angry before meals or when skipping a meal, loss of concentration, restlessness, anxiety, depression, indecision, a craving for sweets or starches (or alcohol), dizziness or weak spells, cold hands and feet, blurred vision, chronic indigestion, and insomnia. There are two primary causes for reactive hypoglycemia: a high intake of refined carbohydrates and food allergies. The first responds well to a diet high in complex carbohydrates—whole grains and legumes. A diet consisting of carbohydrates that turn into sugar slowly is best for both hypoglycemia and diabetes. These are foods which are low in the *glycemic index.*

The glycemic index is one of the most important breakthroughs in blood sugar diets in many years. It has changed the way hypoglycemics and diabetics can eat and yet remain symptom-free. Identified by David Jenkins, M.D., of the University of Toronto, the glycemic index lists the absorption rate of various carbohydrates, showing how fast they turn to sugar. It indicates, for example, that white potatoes turn into sugar more quickly than brown rice, and that pasta is one of the best starches for anyone with a blood sugar handling problem because it turns to sugar slowly.

Added to this, research is being conducted on different forms of food. When a grain or legume is dried and ground into flour, for example, it turns to sugar more quickly than when it is in its natural grain form. This means that whole wheat bread will turn to sugar faster than Tabbouli, a cold, cracked wheat salad (see recipe, chapter 4). Pasta is an exception. All pasta, both whole grain and enriched white, is metabolized slowly. Of course the whole grain varieties contain important nutrients missing in the refined ones, like chromium, a mineral used in blood sugar regulation. Whenever possible, eat whole grain pasta.

The form in which you eat fruit also affects your blood sugar. Fresh, whole fruit turns to sugar more slowly than fruit juice. To liberate sugar (fructose) from an orange, you must first break down the cells that surround it. Since chewing doesn't free all sugar from the fruit (some is broken down by digestive juices in the stomach, other by pancreatic enzymes), the sugar in an orange gets into your bloodstream more slowly than if you drank its juice. Fruit juice contains totally available sugar with no surrounding cellulose. In addition, a four-ounce glass of orange juice may contain the juice—and sugar—from four to six oranges. Eat a piece of fruit instead of drinking fruit juice.

There has been much controversy over the best diet for a hypoglycemic. Some advocate a high-protein, low-carbohydrate program, while others argue for a high complex-carbohydrate, low-protein diet. It is true that protein turns into sugar very slowly, providing energy long after a carbohydrate meal, but it also has a lot of waste products the body has to work hard to eliminate—and high-protein diets have been associated more with disease than health. Diets containing large amounts of complex carbohydrates (whole grains and legumes) have been used to regulate blood sugar conditions for thousands of years. Now under the name "high-fiber diet," some people think it is a new concept. Actually, it is an old, proven way to keep everyone's blood sugar nice and even.

Adult Onset Diabetes: Diabetes brings with it a number of symptoms, including thirst, frequent urination, an increased appetite, weight loss, fatigue, weakness, irritability, cuts that don't heal quickly, poor circulation (numbness and tingling in the feet), and blurred vision.

Adult onset diabetes is frequently accompanied by another symptom: obesity. A poor diet contributes to it, and a good diet low in fats and refined foods is the primary treatment. Stress can cause diabetes later in life as well, but its causes are not clearly understood. Stress-related adult onset diabetes is not related to obesity.

Perhaps the most important dietary information for the overweight person with adult onset diabetes is to keep your calories down and eliminate excess body fat while providing your body with enough vitamins and minerals. This means choosing whole foods low in fats and sugars. Fat slows down the body's ability to utilize sugar, but it's more than twice as high in calories by the gram as either proteins or carbohydrates. Many high-sugar foods are also high in fats.

The diabetic who takes insulin must watch her sugar intake to avoid upsetting the balance it creates. It is best for all diabetics to eat foods low on the glycemic index. If you take insulin, you should be aware of making food exchanges (substituting one permitted food for another). This important and complex subject is adequately covered in other books, such as *The Diabetic's Total Health Book* by June Biermann and Barbara Toohey, and is not repeated here.

Of all the low-fat sugars available, fructose, found in fruit, raises blood sugar most slowly. For this reason, it is the best natural sweetener for diabetics. There is still controversy surrounding such artificial sweeteners as aspartame (Nutrasweet). If you must use an artificial sweetener, use it sparingly. It's best to use fructose in small amounts, thereby reducing your craving for sweets. Fructose, combined with other sweeteners like glucose (in fruit pies and sweetened applesauce, for instance), elevates the blood sugar more quickly than either glucose or fructose by itself, so eat them separately. Make your own pies and tarts with fresh fruit, and eat small quantities of fruit instead of sweetened desserts.

Eliminating the typical desserts will cut down on fats and excess calories. A high-fiber, low-fat diet will help you lose weight and control your diabetes. It will fill you up and help satisfy your desire to eat.

Why the Blood Sugar Diet Works: It eliminates foods that stimulate the insulin response and provides foods that turn into more sugar slowly. It includes information on how often you must eat these foods to stabilize your blood sugar, no matter which type of imbalance you have.

Specifics of the Blood Sugar Diet: The foods eaten by diabetics and hypoglycemics are the same. The amount and frequency of meals differ. Hypoglycemics need to eat frequently, often every four hours. A snack of whole grain crackers or a piece of fresh fruit keeps your energy high and your blood sugar level. If you are trying to lose weight, snack on raw vegetables. Diabetics on a low-calorie regime will do best with three moderate-sized meals a day.

Fat added to a complex carbohydrate slows down the time it takes to turn into sugar. For this reason, you may want to use small amounts of cold-pressed vegetable oil or Better Butter (see recipe, chapter 4) on your pasta, hot cereals, or toast. Whether or not you have a weight problem, keep your fat intake down. Using the Anti-illness Diet as your base, modify as follows:

Eliminate	Reduce	Emphasize
refined sugar	fats	pasta
fruit juices	carrots	non-starchy vegetables like green beans, zucchini, broccoli
dried fruit	parsnips	
white potatoes	fresh corn	beans and lentils
coffee and black tea	yams	brown rice and other whole grains
		herb teas

Pasta is one of the best carbohydrates you can eat. Use whole grain pasta whenever you can, but when you are eating out, white pasta is acceptable. Avoid creamed and butter sauces in favor of tomato-based sauces that are low in fats.

Legumes are another excellent food group to include as a staple. Look for recipes for soup, party dips such as Hummus (see recipe, chapter 4), and hearty side dishes or main courses like chili, tamale pie, and baked beans.

The glycemic index can be helpful for both hypoglycemics and diabetics. By choosing more foods which raise your blood sugar gradually, rather than those that are metabolized more quickly, you can keep your blood sugar even. Following are some suggestions to make this easier, based on higher glycemic foods listed under "Instead of" and lower glycemic foods under "Substitute."

Instead of:	Substitute:
white potatoes	rice, sweet potatoes, or yams
corn flakes	All-Bran, oatmeal, Shredded Wheat
banana	plum, peach, grapefruit, apple, orange
dried fruit	fresh fruit
sugar or honey	fructose
carrots, parsnips	sweet potatoes, yams

Supplements:

Multi-vitamin/mineral two times a day, plus

1000 milligrams vitamin C three times a day, because low vitamin C levels are found in diabetics

15 milligrams zinc, if fatigue may be a result of exhausted adrenal glands. Diabetics excrete more zinc in their urine than other people.

Brewer's yeast—begin with ½ teaspoon and gradually increase to 2 tablespoons per day in cereal or breakfast drink. This is high in chromium, a mineral that works very much like insulin to keep your glucose normal. It may be taken separately in a glucose tolerance factor (GTF) formula, where it is combined with other factors for more efficiency, or as a food in brewer's yeast.

When obesity exists, add the following to help break down fats:

250 milligrams choline three times a day

350 milligrams inositol three times a day

Auxiliary Treatment:

Medical doctor or other health-care practitioner: to monitor your blood sugar and your progress. Choose someone who is familiar with the dietary program you are beginning, so you can communicate with him or her if you have any questions. Often, diabetics using insulin will be able to decrease the amount when they go on a high-fiber diet. Never decrease your medication without first speaking with your doctor.

Exercise: one of the most important additions to a good dietary program. For hypoglycemics, any kind of aerobic exercise, from a brisk twenty-minute walk, to riding a bicycle, swimming, running, or aerobics class, can help your muscles burn fats and eliminate rapid drops in blood sugar. If you can exercise even more, work up to an hour a day and feel the benefits. Diabetics who take insulin should check with their doctors before beginning an exercise program and be certain to eat enough carbohydrates before beginning so they don't run out of blood sugar. For additional information, read *The Diabetic's Total Health Book,* by June Biermann and Barbara Toohey.

THE GOOD DIGESTION DIET

As we have said before, you are not what you eat, but what you digest and absorb. If you don't absorb nutrients into your cells, your body may lack some essential building blocks for good health. When you have deficiencies, your immune system is often weakened, making it more difficult for you to overcome both minor and major illnesses. Fatigued by overproduction of white blood cells to protect you from foreign invaders, the weakened immune system often triggers food allergies. More complete information on each of these subjects is found in the Strong Immune System and the Food Allergy diets in this chapter.

Although there is a direct correlation between good health and good digestion, it is rare to find mention of this association in medical publications. Digestion is overlooked in favor of more complicated solutions. In my practice, I find poor digestion is the beginning of poor health. Restoring the digestive system to a fully functioning system is often the key in reversing illnesses. It is the first, most important step in achieving good health, and a logical place to begin working with your own health.

Without a good digestive system you cannot assimilate the vitamins and minerals from your food. You need ptyalin (an enzyme found in the saliva), hydrochloric acid (HCl, manufactured in the stomach), and pancreatic enzymes. Chewing your food thoroughly is the first step in improving your digestion. This is the first time food is broken down by the teeth on its way to becoming tiny particles of energy. When you taste your food, your taste buds send a message to your brain, identifying it. Then the brain signals your stomach to begin producing hydrochloric acid, needed in the next step of digestion: "Joanna's eating a chicken salad sandwich on rye bread. You had better secrete enough HCl to break this one down!"

The questionnaires in chapter 3 are one way of determining a need for HCl, and having a doctor who understands the importance of having enough HCl in your stomach evaluate your condition is another. If you mistakenly take HCl supplementation and don't need it, you may feel a burning sensation in your stomach. Drinking a glass of water will dilute it and stop the burning. More often than not, we lack sufficient HCl, rather than have too much.

Several factors can inhibit your production of HCl:

1. Age. As we grow older, our stomach produces less HCl. This may be a natural way of keeping us from overeating, since we need less fuel as our metabolism slows down. If you are over 45, your HCl production may already be less than when you were younger, explaining why you can no longer eat everything you used to eat without discomfort.

2. Drinking liquids with meals. Water, coffee, and other liquids dilute HCl in your stomach. This cuts down the available HCl to digest your foods.

3. Drinking cola drinks that contain phosphoric acid. The phosphoric acid tells your stomach that acid is already present, and it does not need to produce HCl.

4. Stress or worry. These reduce enzyme production. If you're upset, don't eat. When you feel you must eat, choose something easy to digest, like a piece of fruit or a piece of whole grain toast. Carbohydrates, which begin digestion in the mouth, are digested faster than proteins.

5. Antacids. They neutralize acids in the stomach that are causing fermentation but also reduce the HCl in your stomach and keep protein from being digested. You may feel better, but you are only treating the symptoms rather than the cause of your discomfort. More HCl, rather than less, is often the solution.

HCl is one of the most important digestive chemicals your body makes. It is responsible for the amount of calcium and iron you absorb, since they both need an acid medium to be utilized. If your stomach is too alkaline (not enough HCl), calcium may collect in your soft tissues instead of getting into your bones. Also, when there isn't enough calcium in your blood, your blood takes what it needs from your bones. All women concerned about getting osteoporosis should be certain they have enough HCl to use the calcium in their food and supplements (see the Osteoporosis Diet). Without enough HCl, iron may not reach your red blood cells, leaving you tired and anemic. In addition, HCl breaks protein down into amino acids for building and repairing muscles.

HCl also triggers the pancreas to produce pancreatic enzymes for the next stage of digestion. If you lack HCl, you may also lack the enzymes you need to further digest your food. In addition to all of this, low HCl production leads to such symptoms as gas, bloating, and indigestion. The best indication that your stomach is not producing enough HCl is the group of symptoms listed in the "Your Current Symptoms" questionnaire under the digestive system section in chapter 3.

Even with adequate HCl production, your body digests different foods at different rates. When you eat protein with carbohydrates, whether they are complex (as in grains) or simple sugars (as in fruit), the carbohydrates are digested first and stay in the stomach while proteins are broken down. Sometimes these carbohydrates ferment, causing gas and heartburn.

Nutritional programs that advocate separating proteins from carbohydrates make a great deal of sense, considering the number of people with digestive problems. In fact, while you are helping your digestive system function better it is a good idea for you to adhere to a low-stress plan of food combining. However, in my opinion the ultimate answer is not to restrict eating enjoyable food combinations, but rather to improve your digestive system so that you can eat, digest, and assimilate almost anything.

Why the Good Digestion Diet Works: It combines a low-stress method of eating (separating proteins from carbohydrates) with HCl and pancreatic enzymes. The supplements give your body the digestive substances it needs to help you digest your food, while the low-stress diet makes digestion easier. By separating foods, you eliminate having some of them fermenting in your stomach and causing gas or bloating.

Specifics of the Good Digestion Diet: The following food-combining information will allow your stomach to digest one kind of food before another one, needing more or less HCl, is eaten:

1. Eat fruit alone.
2. Do not eat proteins with carbohydrates.
3. You may eat proteins with nonstarchy vegetables.
4. You may eat carbohydrates with vegetables.

Vegetarians will not have a problem following these suggestions, since recent information from Frances Moore Lappé, author of *Diet for a Small Planet*, a book on protein combining for vegetarians, indicates food eaten over a twelve-hour period combines in the body to produce complete proteins.

Examples of Proteins	Examples of Carbohydrates
meat, poultry, fish	bread, crackers, chips
cheese, yogurt	potatoes, yams, sweet potatoes
eggs	corn, winter squashes
tofu	all grains
nuts, seeds	legumes
	cookies, cakes
	sugar, honey
	fruit

If you cannot adhere to a strict low-stress diet, modify it by eating smaller amounts of carbohydrates with your proteins or smaller quantities of proteins with your carbohydrates. This is not as easy on your digestive system as separating the two, but it will put less fermentable carbohydrates in your stomach to sit around while proteins are being digested. Examples of lowering your carbohydrate intake with proteins include: an open-faced sandwich with one slice of bread; small amounts of rice with sautéed chicken and vegetables; half a potato with fish or chicken dinners; or eggs with one slice of toast and no potatoes.

Examples of lowering your protein intake with carbohydrates include: two slices of toast with one egg; stir-fried vegetables and rice with a few almonds or slivers of chicken; pasta with a little ground beef, ground turkey, or tofu added to the tomato sauce; tabbouli with a little hummus.

The low-stress diet for good digestion is often difficult for people who need it the most. They frequently eat too fast, don't chew their food well, and eat poor food combinations. If this sounds like you, you can become more aware and slowly change old habits. Here are some suggestions for better food combining:

Instead of:	Substitute:
juice, toast, herb tea	toast, herb tea
eggs, toast, potatoes	vegetable omelet, sliced tomatoes
cereal and fruit	cereal or fruit
chicken, egg, or tuna sandwich	chicken, egg, or tuna salad, hummus or tabbouli with vegetables
meat, chicken, or fish with rice or potatoes and vegetables	meat, chicken, or fish with vegetables, or baked potato and salad, or sautéed or curried vegetables with rice

Better Eating Habits:

1. Follow the food-combining suggestions to the best of your ability.
2. Chew your food thoroughly; taste it.
3. Do not drink liquids with your meals, except wine occasionally, which stimulates the production of HCl.
4. Do not take antacids.

Supplements: B vitamins are needed to produce ptyalin in the mouth and pancreatic enzymes and should be taken daily. Betaine, a factor of vitamin B, is often added to HCl tablets to help stimulate pancreatic enzyme production. After three months, reduce the amount of HCl and enzymes by half. If you get no symptoms within a week or two, gradually reduce them until you take none. Exceptions: if you know you are chronically anemic, continue taking HCl for six months to a year, checking your blood serum iron with your doctor at six-month intervals. When your iron is normal, reduce and eliminate the HCl.

B complex or multi-vitamin/mineral tablet—one to two times a day

150 to 300 grains betaine hydrochloride (HCl) after meals

150 grains betaine hydrochloride (HCl) after snacks, except fruit

60 milligrams pancreatin after meals and snacks, except fruit

Auxiliary Treatment:

Medical doctor: While there are many people who need HCl supplementation, I want to stress the importance of checking this out with a medical doctor or other trained health-care professional. If you have any question about your stomach's ability to produce HCl and your body's ability to manufacture digestive enzymes, have your doctor check it out thoroughly. This can be done through blood tests and other testing methods. If your results are in the lower end of the normal range, you might still benefit from HCl. Ask your doctor if taking it could be harmful in any way. Don't self-medicate.

Chiropractic: Your stomach may not be producing enough HCl because of structural imbalances, such as your spine being out of alignment, which could put pressure on the nerves that bring energy to the stomach. Some cranial faults (bones in the head not perfectly aligned) can cause an underproduction of HCl and are easily corrected by many chiropractors. Ask first if the doctor you speak with is familiar with these techniques.

Acupuncture: Just as drugs can slow down or speed up body functions, so can acupuncture regulate the digestive process, eliminating nausea, belching, and bloating.

THE FATIGUE DIET

Fatigue is a symptom, not a cause. The only way to relieve it is to identify the cause and then eliminate it. There is no Fatigue Diet per se, only clues as to which diet will help you best understand where your problems are coming from and lead you to the diet that will give you more energy.

Fatigue has many sources. It can arise from low amounts of iron in your blood, due to an inadequate intake, or your body's inability to absorb this mineral (see the Good Digestion Diet). It can come from poor digestion, where the foods you eat are not broken down into particles fine enough to enter the cells and provide them with necessary nutrients for energy and repair (see the Good Digestion Diet).

Fatigue can be a result of an allergic reaction—an inability to process a substance (either to digest food or to expel other foreign matter such as pollen, smoke, or other chemicals we inhale). This means eliminating the food allergy whenever possible (see the Food Allergy Diet), strengthening your immune system so it can eradicate the foreign material (see the Strong Immune System Diet), or avoiding the substance. An indication of a food allergy could be tiredness after eating, but since allergic responses can occur from a few minutes to several days afterward, it is not always simple to identify.

When you find yourself getting tired every afternoon, or up to a few hours after eating a lot of sugar or drinking coffee, it may be a sign of a blood sugar imbalance. Both diabetes and hypoglycemia can cause fatigue. Since alcohol is absorbed into the bloodstream quickly, it, too, can cause blood sugar fluctuations and tiredness. Even the nonalcoholic can react to a drink or two when there is a blood sugar handling problem (see the Blood Sugar Diet).

The alcoholic is prone to fatigue, as blood sugar fluctuates with the high sugar intake from the alcohol. The only answer is to stop drinking and begin to repair the body so it can use nutrients from food rather than alcohol as energy. To help stop drinking, the Blood Sugar Diet and AA (Alcoholics Anonymous) are an excellent combination of both physical and emotional support. After you have stopped drinking, the Recovering Alcoholic's Diet can give you strength and increased stamina.

Stress is another factor that can cause fatigue. Whether it is physical, emotional, nutritional, chemical (smog, MSG, exhaust fumes, and so on), gravitational (standing too long), or just plain overwork, you may need to address the cause and slow down. Giving your body a chance to repair itself, getting enough sleep, and adding a minimum of three days of exercise a week (half an hour or more) can eliminate stress-caused fatigue. Psychotherapy, biofeedback, massage, and meditation or relaxation exercises are all excellent daily additions to stress reduction. If you have access to a jacuzzi, use it on a regular basis. If you don't, hot baths are a good alternative. For additional information, see the Stressful Living Diet.

THE HEADACHE DIET

Everyone has headaches from time to time, but chronic headaches are a sign that a health problem exists. They are a symptom, not the problem itself. More common in women than in men, headaches may signal a food or chemical allergy or sensitivity, a response to toxins, fever, inhalation of carbon monoxide, a low-functioning thyroid gland, premenstrual syndrome, the need for food, eye strain or eye dysfunction, tension, or a more complicated condition such as a brain tumor. Many types can be attributed to a sensitivity some people have to a group of chemicals called amines, which are a by-product of certain foods.

You should not "learn to live with" something that may be indicating a problem. If your headache persists after a few simple checks, seek professional help. An osteopath may find you have bones out of alignment that are causing the pain, and a medical doctor who is a headache specialist can suggest brain scans and other tests to reveal hidden problems. Gunnar Heuser, M.D., a headache specialist in Los Angeles, tracked one person's persistent headaches to the way she held the telephone, which caused her neck muscles to cramp.

Headaches are often due to blood vessels that expand or contract too much. Expanded blood vessels set off pain sensors, which results in throbbing as blood is pumped through.

Food Sensitivity Headaches: A number of headaches may originate on your dinner plate. In addition to exploring non-food-related reasons for your recurring pain, you may want to see if changing your diet will eliminate it. Food sensitivity headaches may be from an allergic reaction to a food or the result of a chemical imbalance. With migraines, blood vessels expand too much. When blood cannot pass through these pathways at the rate at which it is being pumped by the heart, blood pressure rises and headaches may occur.

Blood vessels can constrict for a number of reasons, one of which is an increased presence of chemicals called amines. These include tyramine and histamine, which are found in some proteins, and glutamine, present in monosodium glutamate. Allergies can also cause amines to be made, and poor digestion allows them to pass through the wall of the intestines into the bloodstream in increased amounts. If this combination is the cause for your pain, the Food Allergy Diet and the Good Digestion Diet may be your solution.

Some of the most common foods known to cause headaches—milk, wheat, oranges, and chocolate—are all high in amines. If eating a diet high in amine-producing foods is the culprit, you can eliminate them and evaluate the results. Our bodies naturally produce enzymes that break down amines, but these are often found to be missing in people with headaches. According to Dr. Seymour Diamond, president of the National Migraine Foundation, raw spinach may contain this missing enzyme. If amines are causing your discomfort, eliminate as many of them as you can and begin eating a lot of spinach salads.

Foods High in Amines:

aged cheeses	instant and canned soups
alcohol	dry-roasted nuts
chocolate	instant gravy
smoked meats	tenderizers
dairy products	processed meats
pickled foods	MSG
citrus	fermented foods (tofu, soy sauce)

If after a few months you find your headaches respond to a reduced-amine diet, gradually reintroduce foods one at a time, paying close attention to any symptoms they may cause. Keep away from any that invariably cause pain, and monitor the amount of amine-containing foods your body can handle. Try the raw spinach route, eating it for a few weeks and then eliminating it from your diet. With the help of your health diary, you should be able to determine which foods cause problems and how much your body can tolerate of each.

Foods may be your problem, but not necessarily those high in amines. Follow the Food Allergy Diet to eliminate problem foods and perhaps your headaches as well.

Caffeine may be the cause of your headaches. For some people, whose headaches result from enlarged blood vessels, like migraine sufferers, caffeine may eliminate the pain. For others, it is the cause. Caffeine contracts blood vessels going to the brain. Not only is caffeine found in many beverages like coffee, tea, cocoa (and other chocolate products), and cola, but in many headache remedies as well. Read labels carefully and avoid any headache products with caffeine until you are able to eliminate it as a possible originator of your pain.

Caffeine withdrawal headaches are common, as anyone who has given up coffee one or more times knows. This does not mean you should drink more. The pain is a sign your body is addicted to the drug that keeps stimulating it. These headaches disappear in from one to three days, leaving you with a clarity you may have expected from the drug itself. It's easiest to give up coffee on a weekend, when headaches and fatigue don't interfere with the concentration of a busy work schedule.

Insecticides and pesticides are not food, but they enter your body through the foods you eat and become a part of your tissues and can cause headaches. If you are particularly sensitive to these sprays, wash your fruits and vegetables in Clorox. Here is the formula given by Dr. Orion Truss in his book *The Missing Diagnosis:*

Removing insecticides and pesticides: Use only Clorox brand bleach and a stainless steel measuring spoon. Use ½ teaspoon of Clorox for each gallon of water, and place your fruits and vegetables in the solution, using a fresh Clorox bath with each batch of food. The length of time each type of food needs to soak is:

Frozen, leafy vegetables of thin-skin fruits—fifteen minutes.

Thick-skin fruits and root vegetables—twenty minutes.

Thick-skin squash—25 minutes.

Take the fruits and vegetables out of the solution and soak them in clean water for fifteen minutes. They will have no aftertaste, and many people report they stay fresher longer when insecticides and pesticides have been removed in this manner.

Hunger can produce headaches, especially in the person with low blood sugar. If your headaches occur during a time when you've skipped a meal or when you've gone longer than usual without eating, see the Blood Sugar Diet for ways to eliminate the underlying reason. Your brain may not be getting the glucose (blood sugar) it needs to think and may be giving you a signal to feed it.

Migraines. Pain usually occurs on one side of the head at a time and frequently switches to the opposite side. It may be accompanied by nausea, vomiting, and visual disturbances. With migraines, blood vessels become dilated (expanded). Delicate pain sensors are stimulated, producing pain. In more than half the cases there is a family history of migraine, possibly indicating an inherited sensitivity to some foods. There are a number of causes for migraines including stress, fatigue, use of oral contraceptives, and menstruation, but diet is estimated to be a factor in up to 25 percent.

A sensitivity to any food may be causing your migraines if you fall into this category. Following the Food Allergy Diet and eliminating offending foods, along with such alternative therapies as biofeedback (to help you consciously relax) and acupuncture (for relief of pain and to correct imbalances) may produce the long-lasting results you are looking for. A report published in *The Lancet*, a British medical journal, stated that migraine patients were often allergic to food, and most often to three food groups. Pick three to eliminate initially, like dairy products, alcohol, and chocolate.

Since low blood pressure is often present in people with migraines, foods that contain sulfur or other blood pressure–lowering chemicals may be responsible for your headaches, according to Carl Pfeiffer, M.D., biochemical psychiatrist. These include onions, garlic, cabbage, brussel sprouts, chocolate, green peppers, cucumbers, radishes, and watermelon.

Premenstrual Headaches. Palpitating headaches may precede menstruation in women who also suffer from a craving for sweets, increased appetite, heart palpitation, fatigue, and dizziness or fainting. If this describes your headaches, see the Premenstrual Syndrome Diet and follow the recommendations for the elimination of PMT-C.

If, however, your headaches begin about four days after ovulation, or ten days premenstrually, it may be a sign of a hormonal imbalance. According to PMS expert Dr. Guy Abraham, this indication of progesterone elevation and estrogen decline could mean a need for estrogen. See your gynecologist.

Specifics of the Headache Diet: Now that you're more aware of your body and the relationship between what you eat and how you feel, you can select the most likely cause for your headache from the list above. Follow the suggestions given for the category into which you fall. If your headaches do not fit any of these categories, look for additional help from qualified health-care professionals (see Auxiliary Treatment). You can find information on self-help techniques in *Freedom from Headaches*, by Drs. Joel Saper and Kenneth Magee.

Supplements: 100 milligrams niacin for headaches where blood vessels are constricted. Niacin dilates the blood vessels, and works well for these kinds of headaches. In doses over 150 milligrams, niacin may produce flushing, burning, and tingling over your face and upper body. Although this "niacin flush" is not at all harmful, it is not necessary to experience it for niacin to relieve your headache.

Auxiliary Treatment:

Medical Doctor: If you have methodically checked out the alternatives and your headaches persist, see a medical doctor who has a specialty in this area. He or she will be familiar with many causes for headaches and is trained to look in some areas you may have overlooked. If a brain scan is suggested, you may want to follow through to rule out the presence of a tumor—a condition which is often corrected through surgery.

Osteopathic or chiropractic: Misalignments of the spine and cranial bones can cause pressure on nerves, which can lead to many forms of headaches, including migraines. Some chiropractors and osteopaths are familiar with cranial adjustments that can often reduce pressure in the skull. Either kind of practitioner can be helpful when structural imbalances are the cause for your pain.

Acupuncture: Can give immediate pain relief for all kinds of headaches, whether or not they are related to food, and can help correct the underlying causes such as poor digestion, allergies, and tension.

Biofeedback: Can help you control the effect tension has on your body by teaching you to be more aware of how it feels when you are tense and when you're relaxed. By hearing or seeing feedback with the help of a sensitive instrument, you can learn to recognize and control it within yourself without the need for an electronic device.

Meditation/Relaxation Exercises: When headaches are a result of built-up tension, simple relaxation exercises, like watching your breathing for ten minutes, can allow the tension to dissipate. Meditation, or focusing on a single word and saying it to yourself over and over for ten minutes to half an hour, can have similar results. You can use any word, like "love," "peace," "calm," or one which has been used in other cultures and religious practices, like "om." Meditation can be a spiritual/religious experience or a way of reducing tension, or both. Information on books that explain meditation and a cassette that teaches relaxation is found in the beginning of this chapter, under the explanation of Auxiliary Treatments.

Massage: Sometimes a headache is due to accumulated tension, which results in tight neck and shoulder muscles. While it is not a preventive measure, massage can alleviate this pain while you work to reduce stress in your life. For someone who has been experiencing chronic pain, a little pleasure that offers relief is a welcome change.

THE STRONG IMMUNE SYSTEM DIET

I am concerned about the large percentage of my patients of all ages who have weak immune systems. Sometimes detectable only through blood tests until a disease occurs, a strong immunity is one of our most important cornerstones of good health. We are only as healthy as our immune systems, our best protection against aging and disease. The immune system defends us against such foreign invaders as bacteria, malignancy, and partially digested particles of food through the efforts of white blood cells that act somewhat like knights in shining armor.

When you understand how the immune system works, you may be more willing to give it the support it needs now, rather than waiting until colds and flu or a major illness bring it to your attention. Among the white blood cells are T cells and B cells. Think of the T cells as the "transmitters" who send messages to the B cells. The B cells are the "banishers" who do much of the actual work, producing antibodies to destroy unwanted substances. Transmitter and banisher cells are governed by the thymus gland, sometimes called the master gland. The thymus makes hormones that carry its instructions indicating a battle is about to take place to the spleen and lymph nodes, where white blood cells are manufactured and stored. These hormones also gather up the transmitters and send them off to find banisher cells.

Transmitters inform the banishers where foreign invaders are located. They also give messages to another group of white blood cells, the suppressors. These are the "surrounders," with two jobs—to surround and capture invaders and to keep transmitters and banishers from attacking healthy tissue. When there are too few surrounders, healthy organs can be attacked by our own armies. This is what happens in autoimmune diseases like Acquired Immune Deficiency Syndrome (AIDS).

Other things can go wrong with our immune system besides having too few surrounders:

1. A need for specific vitamins and minerals can depress the activity of white blood cells, causing mixed messages to be delivered among transmitters, banishers, and surrounders.

2. Stress can cause our adrenal glands to secrete hormones that reduce the effectiveness of transmitters.

3. Allergies can cause transmitters to become confused so their messages to banishers are not clear. Unable to identify the good guys from the bad guys, banishers go out in a frenzy, overproduce antibodies, and send them off in all directions, frequently destroying healthy tissues and causing allergic reactions. Unchecked, this process can lead to disease in whichever organ the tissues are located, as well as lowered immunity.

4. As we get older, our thymus produces fewer hormones and our armies dwindle at a time when we need them the most. Our immune system becomes less effective with fewer fighters, garbled messages, and haphazard destruction of healthy tissues by misdirected antibodies. Harmful bacteria and viruses can continue unchecked, attacking healthy organs. As a result, our aging accelerates. Organs and healthy tissues not only begin to wear out, our defense system goes haywire and destroys them. There's more breakdown than buildup.

5. Allergies can weaken the immune system by forcing the body to produce more white blood cells when we eat foods we can't completely digest (see the Food Allergy Diet).

You may have a weak immune system if you get frequent colds and flu, if you have chronic allergy symptoms, or if you smoke. Smoking is as harmful to the immune system as it is to the cardiovascular and respiratory systems. Fortunately, its effects on your immunity can usually be reversed within three months after you stop smoking, according to research published in the *International Clinical Nutrition Review* in April, 1984. You want to strengthen your defense mechanisms if any of these conditions are present, if there is a history of cancer in your family, or if you are interested in slowing down the aging process.

The vitamins needed by a strong immune system include some of the B vitamins, particularly B_6, B_{12}, and folic acid. They stabilize transmitter response. B_6 also stabilizes banishers and the hormone activity of the thymus, and both B_6 and pantothenic acid are needed to make antibodies. Many multivitamins are rather low in B_6. Some designed for premenstrual syndrome contain larger amounts to eliminate edema. I have found them to be preferable to a general B complex.

A great deal has been noted in health literature about the effects of vitamin C to help fight infections and keep an immune system strong. It is also used for the production of antibodies. There is good reason to take rather large amounts of vitamin C while building a stronger defense system. I have seen beneficial results from taking megadoses of this vitamin for a number of complaints, from colds to bladder infections; the only exception is that large doses of C may produce kidney stones in people with gout.

You need enough vitamin A, and this is usually found in abundance in fresh fruits and vegetables, as well as multivitamin tablets. High doses of vitamin A have been found to enhance the work of banishers but should be administered by a health-care professional who has determined your body's ability to handle it. It is an oil-soluble vitamin that the body stores and can be toxic in large amounts.

Both vitamin E and selenium, found in vegetable oils and brewer's yeast, are required for a strong immune system, but an experiment reported in *The Journal of the American Medical Association* indicated too much E depressed the immune system in healthy people. I have spoken with several biochemists who agree with this information, and suggest vitamin E be taken in no more than 1000 iu a day. I prefer to be a little more conservative. For this reason, if you suspect you have an immune deficiency, I suggest you take a maximum of 800 iu of vitamin E a day, which is the same amount suggested by many gynecologists to reduce or eliminate breast cysts.

You need the right amount of fats—enough essential fatty acids (found in cold-pressed vegetable oils), and enough cholesterol, manufactured by a healthy liver, to nourish your white blood cells. If you don't have enough cholesterol, you end up with weak, hungry transmitters and banishers. An abnormally low cholesterol level is an indication your immune system is also low. Too much cholesterol, on the other hand, leads to immune suppression. If you have a recent blood test, look at your cholesterol. Ideally, I agree with those cardiologists who believe it should be somewhere between 160 and 190 milligrams.

Both iron and zinc can be harmful in excess, but both are needed for a healthy immune system. Unless a health-care practitioner tells you that your body needs more, a multi-vitamin/mineral tablet will prevent a deficiency.

Some substances are a strain on the immune system. Aspirin, for example, suppresses the transmitters. If you need a pain killer, many health food stores carry some made from white willow bark. The active ingredient in aspirin is the synthetic derivative of white willow bark—salicylate. Alcohol and recreational drugs (marijuana, cocaine, and so on) are counterproductive to building a healthy immune system. You may be able to tolerate a few drinks when you're stronger, but avoid it for now, along with any other substances that don't add to your health.

Why the Strong Immune System Diet Works: The best diet for a strong immune system is the Anti-illness Diet, with a few added supplements and recommendations. It provides you with the vitamins and minerals needed to nourish your white blood cells so they can send messages, make antibodies, and destroy only the harmful invaders.

Specifics of the Strong Immune System Diet: According to Roy L. Walford, M.D., UCLA gerontologist and author of *Maximum Life Span*, eating small quantities of food puts less of a stress on the immune system and actually leads to its rejuvenation. Keep your portions small, and don't eat when you're not hungry. To prevent your immune system from working overtime destroying partially digested particles of food, you would be wise to refer to the Food Allergy Diet and the Good Digestion Diet. If it sounds as though either of them apply to you, follow it for a minimum of three months.

Eliminate	Reduce	Emphasize
cigarettes	amount of food you eat	fresh fruits
alcohol	fats	fresh vegetables
drugs		whole grains
aspirin		

Supplements: Eliminating vitamin and mineral deficiencies and improving your diet can strengthen your immunity. Taking supplements containing raw whole thymus gland is thought by many practitioners to help rejuvenate the thymus, which is said to lose 80 percent to 90 percent of its ability to handle toxins and fight invaders as we age.

Multi-vitamin/mineral with high levels of B_6, like Optivite

1000 milligrams vitamin C, three to six times a day

400 iu water-soluble vitamin E, two times a day

200 to 400 milligrams whole raw thymus gland (found in health food stores) three times a day

Auxiliary Treatments:

Acupuncture: Strengthens the immune system by increasing circulation and red blood cell production, promoting optimal functioning of all organs.

Massage: Promotes circulation throughout the body and helps drain the lymphatic system, which carries debris from the white blood cells out of the body via the urine.

Stress reduction: Swimming, jogging, yoga, or any forms of exercise to reduce stress can prevent production of adrenal gland hormones that weaken the system. Meditation or relaxation exercises once or twice a day can help you cope more easily with daily stresses, and biofeedback can help you identify and lower stress.

THE HEALTHY SKIN DIET

Your skin is the largest organ of the body. It has two functions: to protect delicate tissues from being exposed to dirt, bacteria, and the elements; and to eliminate toxins not disposed of through the kidneys and colon. Your skin condition tells you several things about your body. It lets you know how well you're eliminating wastes, and it may indicate a need for specific vitamins. Some skin problems are caused by an accumulation of waste products that have no other way to leave the body. Boils and blemishes are examples of a need for internal cleansing. A change of diet and an increase in water intake frequently can eliminate these problems. As for vitamins, dry skin, acne, dermatitis (like eczema), and even wrinkles may be your body's way of asking for vitamin A, vitamin E, biotin, niacin, zinc, or essential fatty acids.

Many skin problems can be helped with a diet that avoids fried foods, refined foods, caffeine, alcohol, additives, and preservatives. Since your body can't use them for growth or repair, it must eliminate them. Daily servings of fresh fruits and vegetables and whole grains supply some of the vitamins and minerals needed for healthy skin, while nuts, seeds, and cold-pressed vegetable oils give it essential fatty acids for moisture. The first thing I do with a patient who has skin problems is put them on the Anti-illness diet. It is often the last thing I have to do as well.

A good diet, however, may not be sufficient if you have a skin problem that is the result of having too little vitamin A, not enough essential fatty acids, or fat malabsorption. You may be eating enough of the right foods, but unable to get the nutrients into your cells. Fat malabsorption is a common problem, caused by a lack of pancreatic enzymes that, along with bile, breaks down fat-soluble vitamins. It may be caused by food allergies, which can produce an inflammation in the cells of the small intestines, where most nutrients are absorbed. Refer to the Food Allergy Diet and the Good Digestion Diet for further information if you believe they may apply to you.

Acne. There are many theories concerning the control and elimination of acne, including eating a diet free of sugar, chocolate, and fried foods. While such a diet can contribute to healthier skin, it has not been proven effective in getting rid of this stubborn condition. John Kirschmann, in *Nutrition Almanac*, reports success with niacin, one of the B vitamins. In a test where twenty people were given niacin supplementation, it brought relief to every one. In addition to cleaning up your diet, it is worth trying niacin, which has no side effects.

Dermatitis. Skin inflammation can come from allergies to foods or airborne irritants. It is often aggravated by fatigue or stress. When this is the case, the best solution is to avoid the food that causes a reaction and follow the Food Allergy Diet. Supplements listed in that diet help strengthen the body's natural defenses against both food and airborne allergies. Moreover, some vitamins and minerals can be useful in cases of dermatitis. Biotin, one of the B vitamins, is one of these. *Nutrition Almanac* cites a report published in the *Journal of Pediatrics* that found biotin tablets to be effective in mild cases of dermatitis and biotin injections helpful in more severe instances. You may want to speak with your doctor about using this approach.

Zinc is a mineral used to heal a variety of skin problems, including dermatitis. One sign of a zinc deficiency is the presence of white spots on the fingernails. If you have these white spots, take zinc until the initial spots have grown out and you can see no more have appeared, then discontinue them since too much zinc could cause a copper deficiency. Zinc is needed by ribonucleic acid, a substance found in all cells that gives instructions to repair skin and other tissues. To be absorbed, zinc needs enough pancreatic enzymes. Because your digestive system may be involved, refer to the Good Digestion Diet before supplementing with zinc or adding pancreatic enzymes to your program.

Dry skin. Rough, dry skin often signals a need for vitamin A, which helps repair all tissues and keeps the skin smooth and soft. Vitamin A is found in abundance in many fresh fruits and vegetables (especially in those that are yellow, orange, red, or dark green and leafy). Even if you are eating these foods regularly, however, you may not be absorbing vitamin A if you have digestive problems. Poor digestion often means a difficulty in absorbing fat-soluble vitamins. For this reason, be certain the supplement you take is in a water-soluble tablet or an emulsified liquid, rather than an oil-based capsule, for easier, more complete assimilation.

Dry skin may also indicate a need for essential fatty acids, found in nuts and seeds, foods many women avoid because they are thought to be fattening and tend to be difficult to digest. Essential fatty acids are also found in vegetable, seed, and nut oils, like safflower and sesame oils. EFAs are destroyed by heat, so nuts and seeds must be raw to contain them, and the oils cold-pressed. To prevent these oils from becoming rancid in the body and damaging cells, even if they're not rancid when ingested, essential fatty acids should be accompanied by vitamin E, which counteracts this effect.

Wrinkles. While wrinkles may be inevitable, there's no need to rush them. Heredity may play a part in how fast you age, as does smoking and alcohol. There's not much you can do about heredity, but you can control how long you bake in the sun. Constant exposure to the sun's rays dries out your skin, contributing to wrinkles. Wear sunscreen, moisturize your skin after exposure, and limit sun-bathing to cut down on wrinkles and lower your chances of getting skin cancer as well. Lubricate your skin from the inside out by including cold-pressed vegetable oils in your diet to give your skin the essential fatty acids it needs to remain smooth and flexible.

Hormone imbalance can contribute to loss of skin elasticity and wrinkling. Estrogen causes skin to become less elastic and progesterone helps keep it firm. A number of conditions, including aging and premenstrual syndrome can contribute to lowered progesterone levels, and some supplements are effective in raising them. I have seen the dramatic effects of Optivite on progesterone levels in a nine-month study I conducted under the direction of Dr. Guy Abraham, who designed the supplement. In this study on liver function and hormone levels in women with PMS, progesterone levels were below normal when the study began, and normal after taking vitamin and mineral supplementation for six months. I only have experience with this particular formula and do not know whether or not others are as effectively absorbed and will give similar results, but you may want to try this approach for healthier skin instead of taking hormones. You can also include more eggs and sweet potatoes in your diet, since both have been found to contain natural progesterone.

Why the Healthy Skin Diet Works: It consists of whole foods filled with vitamins and nutrients both for the skin and other organs. This prevents vitamin and mineral deficiencies from occurring in the future that may directly affect your skin problems. It also assures that most of what you eat is used to nourish cells, leaving fewer toxic substances to be identified, sorted out, and eliminated. You are more likely to get rid of wastes through the kidneys and colon when they are not overworked and when you flush out wastes with plenty of water. This diet is high in such roughage as whole grains, fresh vegetables, and fruit to prevent constipation and shorten the time it takes solid wastes to leave the body.

Specifics of the Healthy Skin Diet: Use the Anti-illness Diet as the basis for your nutritional program, with an emphasis on fresh vegetables and copious amounts of water. Drink pure water throughout the day in small quantities (four ounces an hour whenever possible) to help eliminate wastes through the urine and prevent constipation.

Type of Condition	Eliminate	Reduce	Emphasize
all skin problems	fats		water
	refined foods		roughage (whole grains, fruits, and vegetables)
	caffeine		
	alcohol		
	chocolate		
	fried foods		
wrinkles			eggs
			sweet potatoes
dry skin			fresh fruits and vegetables
			cold-pressed vegetable oils

Supplements:

Acne:
100 milligrams niacin three times a day for three weeks, or until you experience a regular flushing

Dermatitis:
1 milligram (not microgram) biotin, three to four times a day
50 milligrams zinc three times a day for one to two months. High doses of zinc can decrease the copper in your system. Don't use large amounts for longer without a doctor's supervision.

Dry skin:
25,000 iu dry or emulsified vitamin A, two times a day
1 to 2 tablespoons of cold-pressed safflower oil
100 to 200 iu dry vitamin E

Wrinkles:
6 Optivite tablets a day to normalize progesterone

Auxiliary Treatment:

Exercise: Aerobic exercise stimulates circulation throughout the body, increasing elimination. A brisk half-hour walk, a run around the high school track, tennis, racquetball, or swimming are all excellent exercises for improving the function of your colon and the condition of your skin.

Steam Room: If you have access to a steam room in a health spa, use it to increase your detoxification. Drink plenty of water before and after you steam to prevent dehydration. For healthy skin, always use wet heat, rather than dry. When asked whether a steam or sauna was best, one skin-care specialist replied, "Steam, without a doubt. If you go into a sauna, be sure to take a chicken with you. When it's cooked, you will be, too." Dry heat is like an oven, while steam moisturizes. Always rinse your face with cool water afterward to close pores that steam or hot water have opened.

DIETS FOR THE ABCs OF EATING

Food is not the cause of eating disorders. If you have anorexia, bulimia, or eat compulsively, you use food to avoid dealing with psychological problems. Eating disorders frequently stem from unresolved emotional problems and require the understanding that comes from individual or group counseling before they can be eliminated. Therapists who have sent patients to me for a nutritional workup find the combination of nutritional and psychological counseling shortens both therapies. You may be the rare individual who can be helped with nutrition alone. However, if you are not, don't hesitate to seek help with a therapist who understands the importance of good nutrition.

THE ANOREXIA DIET

Anorexia, discovered in 1689 by an English doctor, Richard Morton, has come out in the open during the past few years. It is a form of self-starvation affecting ten to twenty times more women than men. Anorexia often begins when a woman is in her teens or early twenties. Most typically, the anorectic comes from an upper-middle-class family with a dominating mother who emphasizes thinness. The mother often has some form of eating disorder as well. Anorexia is one way the young woman can have control over both her mother and her own life, by rigidly monitoring her weight. Along with eating too little, she may spend hours each day exercising vigorously in a further attempt to maintain control and lose more weight.

She sees herself in a distorted light, thinking herself fat while others see her as gaunt and emaciated. Her head is frequently larger in proportion to the rest of her body, which has matchstick arms and legs. In addition to thinking of herself as being overweight, the anorectic has so much willpower over food she frequently cannot identify hunger. She is obsessed with food, often preparing it for others, and may even know a great deal about its caloric, vitamin, and mineral values. Unlike other forms of malnutrition, the anorectic is not likely to have a protein deficiency, although a protein deficiency may occur in some cases. Since protein does not contribute to weight gain, except when eaten in excess, she views it as one of the safer foods.

Despite sufficient protein, the anorectic loses muscle tissue. Weight loss of at least 25 percent of original body weight is a sign of anorexia, and as weight is lost, fat is burned for energy. When there is no more fat to burn, the body feeds off muscles, eating itself up and causing a loss of muscle tone and weakness. With little protective fat to shield against the elements, the anorectic is often cold, even in warm climates. Other health problems that are a direct result of anorexia include fluid retention, anemia, gastrointestinal problems, amenorrhea (lack of menstruation), constipation, dry skin, and brittle hair and nails—some of which are signs of hormonal imbalances.

Anorexia is the most difficult of all eating disorders to treat since the anorectic does not believe there is anything wrong with herself. Her knowledge of vitamins and minerals may give her the false impression she is giving herself all the essential nutrients to be healthy, but she tends to omit important foods by eliminating grains, nuts, and oils. David Horrobin, M.D., pioneer in the field of essential fatty acids, believes anorexia is due to a deficiency of zinc and EFAs. Zinc, found in oatmeal, nuts, corn, and pumpkin seeds, is needed for EFA metabolism, and EFAs found in cold-pressed vegetable oils are needed for zinc absorption. Each is dependent on the other, and the anorectic's diet is often lacking in both.

An article in *The Lancet* substantiates the presence of a zinc deficiency in anorexia. Zinc is excreted more rapidly in starvation. Since it contributes to our ability to taste and smell, a zinc deficiency is accompanied by a decreased desire for food. An anorectic who has little taste for food might do well to supplement her diet with zinc.

Most people afraid of gaining weight are not afraid of gaining muscle tone and filling out a thin neck and arms. They are worried about heavy thighs and a protruding belly. The latter is sometimes a result of poor digestion, and the former may signal a need for daily walking, running, or other leg exercises. The anorectic who is concerned about a distended stomach should read the Good Digestion Diet. Her condition may be due to incomplete digestion, or it may be a misperception. Her stomach may not be distended at all, except in her mind.

If you have been told by a number of people that you are too thin, if you don't eat regular meals and work to keep your weight down by restricting your diet and/or by exercising, if your menstruation has stopped and you have other signs of anorexia, check out your condition with a qualified therapist. Therapy will help you understand whether or not you have this type of eating disorder, and if so, how to preserve your health.

Why the Anorexia Diet Works: It emphasizes eating small quantities of food throughout the day and provides some of the nutrients typically missing from this type of reducing diet. Essential fatty acids, replaced by adding a little cold-pressed vegetable oils to salad dressing, may normalize the hormonal balance when a deficiency contributed to its cause. It provides whole grains, to supply heat and energy, so muscles will not become wasted and body temperature will feel more comfortable.

Specifics of the Anorexia Diet: Most problems resulting from anorexia, including endocrine imbalances that cause hormonal imbalances, disappear with sufficient weight gain. An understanding of how you are harming your body instead of keeping it as strong and healthy as you believe may help you become willing to eat a little more and exercise a little less. Weight gain may simply be a result of rebuilding muscles, not storing excess fat. Since your food intake tends to be limited, you need high-quality foods at all times. Eat small amounts of whole foods throughout the day. It is important for you to eat enough food to supply your body with the nutrients it needs for good health. This means eating more than you have been eating, but by concentrating on nutritious foods, you can regain your health without eating large quantities.

Eliminate	Reduce	Emphasize
refined foods		1 tablespoon cold-pressed safflower oil daily in salad dressing
		small amounts of Better Butter (see chapter 4)
		whole grains

Supplements:

Multi-vitamin/mineral

15 milligrams zinc three times daily after food for one month. Since an excess can upset the zinc and copper balances in your body, do not continue taking zinc unless you are under a doctor's care.

THE BULIMIA AND COMPULSIVE-EATING DIET:

Bulimia. Some anorectics are bulimic, but not all bulimics are anorectic. Bulimia consists of eating normally, then binging, usually on "forbidden" foods high in sugar or fats. This is followed by purging with laxatives, diuretics, or self-induced vomiting. Depression and low self-esteem often accompany the binge-purge syndrome. While an anorectic is easily identified by her appearance, bulimics come in all ages and sizes. They are so secretive that they manage to hide their condition from close friends and family members. Afraid of not being able to stop their binges, purging is their answer to an out-of-control situation.

Sometimes the bulimic craves certain foods, which may indicate a food allergy or blood sugar imbalance. Sometimes it is their body asking for a specific nutrient. Often, however, a bulimic is trying to fill an emotional emptiness with food, which provides only temporary satisfaction.

In addition, continual purging causes metabolic imbalances. A Russian study comparing anorectics with bulimics showed cholesterol, potassium, sodium, and calcium were below normal in bulimics and not in anorectics. Sodium and potassium are electrolytes, atoms needed along with fluids in the proper balance for nerve and muscle function. When this balance is upset, serious conditions can result, including abdominal pain, fatigue, headaches, heart palpitations, kidney dysfunctions, and muscle weakness.

Vomiting leads to dehydration and a loss of potassium. Calcium absorption, dependent upon sufficient hydrochloric acid in the stomach, may be prevented as HC1 is regurgitated into the mouth. This can lead to premenstrual syndrome and osteoporosis, as pointed out in the Premenstrual Syndrome Diet and the Osteoporosis Diet. Powerful gastric jucies in the mouth can wear enamel off teeth, and constant vomiting can cause a sore or bleeding throat, swollen and infected salivary glands, and chronic indigestion.

Using laxatives to get rid of excess foods is both senseless and harmful. It is senseless because by the time your digestive acids and enzymes have mixed with food and the food has reached your colon, it has already been in your small intestines, where its nutrients are absorbed. Whatever is going to be utilized has been utilized. All laxatives do is speed up the time it takes waste products to leave your body and create dehydration, since water is absorbed through the colon.

Excessive use of laxatives—besides upsetting the electrolyte balance with the results previously mentioned—can also cause a cathartic (or laxative) colon, which means your colon becomes a tube with no peristaltic action. Peristalsis is the series of small wavelike intestinal contractions that push wastes along. Without it, you become dependent upon laxatives to have regular bowel movements. Diuretics are not the answer, either; they upset the potassium level and leave you constipated, while your kidneys work overtime to eliminate the water your body needs.

When a bulimic seeks help she is concerned about her health or is ready to stop hiding and give up an uncomfortable and expensive habit. Since she uses purging to get rid of forbidden foods or foods eaten in excess, the first lesson to learn is that nothing is forbidden. There are only some foods which are better than others.

Compulsive Eating. Compulsive overeaters have similar emotional patterns to bulimics but do not purge themselves after binging. Both may binge continuously, usually when they feel worthless or under stress, and both feel like failures each time they succumb. Overeating is a way to avoid sexual feelings and interactions, to avoid anger, and to remain passive. You may be eating compulsively to avoid a feeling or to fill a void. If the emptiness is emotional, food won't fill it. It can only fill a physical emptiness, like physical hunger. Emotional spaces are filled with emotions and understanding. Use a combination of therapy and a better understanding of nutrition to overcome this pattern.

In addition to psychological reasons for eating there may be biochemical ones. Since food allergies may be a cause, refer to the Food Allergy Diet for further information, or try eating a few more carbohydrates if you have cut down on them. Judith Wurtman, a nutrition research scientist at the Massachusetts Institute of Technology, found some people who craved carbohydrates were actually listening to their bodies. Their brains were asking for serotonin, a chemical that causes blood vessels to dilate and contract. Wurtman believes serotonin may make people feel more relaxed. When she added a small carbohydrate snack to the diets of carbohydrate cravers they became calmer, the craving left, and many were able to lose weight.

Your body may be asking for particular foods. If you are a compulsive overeater you are probably not listening closely to it or not hearing when it's had enough. By focusing on your body, rather than your emotions, you can overcome automatic eating. Compulsive eaters are afraid of food and the power it has over them.

Why the Bulimia and Compulsive-Eating Diet Works: It provides you with alternatives to your eating patterns that allow you to break the cycle and view food differently. It places the emphasis where it belongs: on the emotional causes for your physical problem.

Specifics of the Bulimia and Compulsive-Eating Diet: Food has no power except whatever power you give it. Take this power back into your own hands. The following suggestions have worked successfully for many of my patients. They have been designed to help you stop binging and feeling like a failure. All of them may not work for you, but if one suggestion takes you a step closer to moving past your eating disorder, its purpose has been served.

1. There are no forbidden foods. If you give yourself the precise food you want when you want it, you will satisfy your urge for it. If you want a piece of cake, don't eat a sandwich, fruit, chips, a salad, and a few rolls in your attempt to avoid the cake. Eat what you want, but only as much as you want to satisfy your desire. If you cannot control the amount you eat, go to the next suggestion.

2. Use the "better than" approach. Some foods are better than others. Whole, unrefined, unprocessed foods are best. Even though there are no forbidden foods, be aware of what you are eating and choose something

that is better than what you would choose ordinarily. A piece of fruit is better than a brownie if you are able to make that choice. Half a brownie is better than a whole one if you're not.

3. When you "blow it," you blow it only in that moment. Going off whatever program you are on doesn't give you permission to overeat the rest of the day or week. Move past your all-or-nothing position. Stay on your program whenever possible, and when you go off it, get back on it right away. Be more careful instead of guilty, angry, or upset.

4. Be aware of hunger. Eat when you're hungry and eat only enough to take away your hunger and let you still feel comfortable. Don't eat until you feel stuffed. Feeling full is your stomach's way of saying, "I'm near my limits." Whatever you would enjoy eating when you're full will taste even better the next time you're hungry. Save it.

5. Experience hunger at least a few times a week, unless you have a blood sugar problem. Enjoy the feeling for a few minutes to an hour before eating. Become comfortable with hunger, realizing you can always eat and get rid of it. When you're hungry, your body is eating your fat for energy, instead of using food. This is how you lose weight.

6. Make an "alternatives to eating" list. When you are feeling emotionally empty, what could you do instead of eat? Make a list of everything from calling a friend, taking a walk, reading a magazine, or going to a movie to asking for a hug or taking a relaxing bath with candlelight and music in the background. If putting something in your stomach is the only solution, make a pot of chamomile or other herb tea, and drink away until your heart (and body) is content.

Auxiliary Treatment:

Therapy: Find a therapist or a group therapy situation that deals with eating disorders and start understanding where the part of you that uses food to destroy rather than nourish comes from. A rigid food program that tells you which foods you're allowed deals only with your symptoms. It will not help you solve your problem. You will be dieting forever. Instead, use a combination of counseling and new eating habits to get to the cause and to bring you satisfying solutions. Then you will be in charge of your life and can move beyond the programming you received that resulted in your eating disorder.

If you don't know where to turn to, you can write or phone the following organizations which publish newsletters that include information on educational programs across the country:

ANRED (Anorexia Nervosa and Related Eating Disorders, Inc.)
P.O. Box 5102
Eugene, OR. 97405
(503) 344–1144
$5 newsletter subscription

American Anorexia Nervosa Association
133 Cedar Lane
Teaneck, N.J. 07666
(201) 836–1800 10 A.M.–2 P.M. Eastern Standard Time

For a list of institutions across the country with programs on eating disorders, and other pertinent information, write to:

Carole Edelstein, M.D.
UCLA Eating Disorders Program
Neuropsychiatric Institute
760 Westwood Plaza
Los Angeles, CA. 90024

Exercise: Some people eat when they are bored. Moderate exercise takes away the appetite and gets you away from food. If you find exercise boring, at least it prevents you from being bored in front of the television set where you can eat. It's better to be bored at a gym or taking a walk with a friend than near the refrigerator. Exercise will help you burn up more calories and firm up muscles as well. Use it, but don't abuse your body by overexercising. Half an hour to an hour a day is plenty to get positive results.

Relaxation or meditation: Eating disorders are stressful and come from emotional stresses that can be reduced through meditation or relaxation techniques. One effective method is to close your eyes and cup your hands together in front of you. Think of all the love you feel for various people in your life. Think of all the love these people have for you. If you cannot feel love, feel the loveliness and beauty of a sunset or a bouquet of flowers. Feel this so clearly you can feel it grow warm and heavy in your hands. When you are holding all the love or beauty you can, place your hands over your stomach and feel it seep in, filling you. Whatever love you need you can give yourself. You can fill yourself with the beauty in nature and be nourished.

Other suggestions for books and tapes that teach relaxation and meditation techniques are given in the beginning of this chapter under the description of Auxiliary Treatments.

DIETS FOR THE REPRODUCTIVE SYSTEM

THE AMENORRHEA DIET

Amenorrhea is a condition in which a woman either stops or does not begin menstruating. Although some women consider it a convenience, the hormones produced during the menstrual cycle contribute to our health and a lack of them can cause problems. Primary amenorrhea is defined as a condition in which menstruation does not begin by age eighteen. This can be caused by genetic abnormalities, malfunctions of the pituitary, ovarian or adrenal tumors, delayed puberty, malnutrition, or anorexia. Any woman who has not begun menstruating by this time should be evaluated by a gynecologist.

Secondary amenorrhea occurs after menstruation has begun when your hormone production has become upset due to severe dietary changes, stress, or excessive exercise. In some cases of amenorrhea, the body doesn't manufacture estrogen, which increases the risk of osteoporosis (see the Osteoporosis Diet). In other cases, the body produces estrogen, but not progesterone. We need both estrogen (to prevent osteoporosis and to stimulate the lining of the uterus) and progesterone (to prevent this lining from growing too rapidly, resulting in a cancerous condition).

Secondary amenorrhea can be caused by a variety of circumstances, from low body fat and excessive exercise to more serious conditions such as an underactive thyroid, premature menopause, or a pituitary gland tumor. It is important to explore the reasons for amenorrhea to rule out thyroid problems or tumors, which require medical attention, before you decide that diet alone will help you. In addition to diet, there are other avenues for the amenorrheic woman to explore: stress reduction techniques, modifying an exercise regime, acupuncture, and chiropractic treatments have all been found effective.

Low body fat and overexercising can result from a preoccupation with dieting and keeping in shape, or they can occur in the professional or amateur athlete who has a rigorous training schedule. The danger in either is in going too far. The exercise boom which blossomed in the early 1980s has led to exercise-associated amenorrhea caused by low body fat in distance runners, swimmers, bodybuilders, and professional dancers. Low body fat is associated with hormonal changes, which can result in irregular menstruation or amenorrhea.

Competitive stress may contribute to amenorrhea in people who over-exercise. Both stress and strenuous exercise produce beta-endorphins, hormones that can make you feel so good after a strenuous workout you might forget the pain of pushing muscles to their limit. Endorphins can slow down the release of other hormones and cause decreased estrogen production, leading to amenor-rhea. It is important to understand that your exercise routine may be contributing to your problem, while a modified workout could give you the results you are looking for in sports and allow your body to function more normally.

Both low-fat and total vegetarian diets are another possible cause. In an article in *The Lancet,* a British medical journal, low-fat and vegetarian diets were said to influence both the amount of estrogen the body makes and how much it excretes. If not enough is manufactured, or if too much is eliminated, the result is low blood estrogen—a precursor of amenorrhea.

Another type of amenorrhea can be produced by a particular kind of vegeta-rian diet—one that contains large quantities of carrots and other vegetables high in carotene (broccoli, spinach, pumpkins, and squash). This form of amenorrhea is easily corrected. An article in the *Journal of the American Medical Association* reports a study in which every one of the women ate more protein and reduced their intake of carotene, and began menstruating within a few months. These women were all healthy, of normal weight, and did not exercise strenuously. Their one common factor was a diet high in vegetables containing carotene. In support of this theory, pills containing carotene, which were sold in Europe to help people tan faster, were found to lead to menstrual disorders when they were used excessively.

Small amounts of fats and a little protein seem to be essential in reversing amenorrhea. However, some people don't eat much protein because they claim they don't like it. It may actually be that their stomachs are not producing enough hydrochloric acid to digest meat and other proteins. If you have amenorrhea and are not attracted to eating protein, explore your body's ability to digest it before increasing the amount you eat (refer to the Good Digestion Diet).

Weight gain is often sufficient to reverse amenorrhea, even when the thyroid level is low. *Postgraduate Medical Journal,* an English publication, reports that amenorrhea can be eliminated and low thyroids normalize themselves when weight is increased.

Sometimes, however, there is no simple answer. In an effort to find workable solutions I have explored less traditional methods, such as acupuncture and

Oriental medicine. In some cases I have found them to be quite effective. Oriental medicine examines the whole system whenever a problem exists, not just the localized area, such as the reproductive system. In a number of cases where body fat was normal, stress and exercise were reduced, there were no clinical abnormalities, and no sign of menstruation was evident, Oriental medicine provided me with the additional information I needed to help women overcome their amenorrhea through diet.

In Oriental medicine, amenorrhea and other gynecological problems are said to come from blood congestion or a "coldness" in the body. This view is quite compatible with a more conventional Western stance. It is well-known that some foods—such as fruits, vegetables, and dairy products—keep the body cool while others produce heat. This is why we tend to eat a lot of salads and fruit and drink lemonade in the summer, and eat starchier vegetables and potatoes in winter.

Laura was twenty-six when she first came to see me. Her period had stopped a year and a half before when she took major exams in school. The year prior, they had been irregular. Her diet included large amounts of fruit, salads, and yogurt, all cooling foods. I asked Laura to begin adding whole grains, ginger tea, and miso soup to her meals. Miso, a soy bean paste, can be added to soups for flavor, and heats the body from the inside out. Laura made miso soup often, and began eating more curried foods for dinner. Her period began within two months and continues to be regular. She still includes some warming foods and spices in her diet.

With *all* women who have amenorrhea, I suggest a diet high in heat-producing foods (whole grains, protein, miso soup, and some spices like ginger and cayenne). You can drink ginger tea, made by pan-roasting either fresh or dried pieces of ginger root, then boiling the root for five or ten minutes. At the same time, reduce the amount of cooling foods, especially salads, fruit, and cold meals. I have found excellent results using this diet. In a number of cases, menstruation began within a month or two and continued to be normal.

Why the Amenorrhea Diet Works: Not all amenorrhea will be reversed by this or any other nutritional program. Some cases of amenorrhea are persistent even in the face of excellent medical, nutritional, and alternative-care treatments. Depending on the type of amenorrhea you have, dietary changes can increase your body weight to normal, give you needed nutrients for a balanced menstrual cycle, and eliminate problem foods that could be causing the imbalance. The Anti-illness Diet may not be sufficient if you are choosing to eat cooling foods, little or no fats, not enough protein, and if you persist in overexercising. The same foods, eaten in another form (cooked or with some spices added), may be all you need—or it may be necessary to make some specific modifications to get the results you're looking for.

Specifics of the Amenorrhea Diet: Since amenorrhea may come from a number of reasons, first determine the cause that applies most closely to you, then add the recommended changes to your Anti-illness Diet.

Supplements: If you have not been eating much protein and notice a feeling of heaviness after you eat it, you may need HCl. Refer to the Good Digestion Diet to assist you in getting the specific supplement you need before buying digestive aids. If you have been a lacto-ovo vegetarian, you may lack vitamin B_{12}. Rather

Type	Eliminate	Reduce	Emphasize
low body fat			some vegetable oils more food
heavy exercising or stress			whole grains some vegetable oils
low-fat or vegetarian diet			some vegetable oils more combined protein (grains and legumes)
high-carotene diet	carrots, broccoli, spinach, pumpkins, squash		more protein
blood congestion or coldness in body	raw fruits and vegetables	cooked vegetables cold foods dairy	whole grains protein miso soup ginger tea spices: cayenne, curry powder, ginger cooked foods

than take this vitamin by itself, take a complete B-complex for a more balanced supplement.

HCl if needed to help digest protein

B-complex if you have been a total vegetarian

Auxiliary Treatment:

Medical doctor: To rule out thyroid problems, tumors, or other causes for amenorrhea that may need medical attention. Follow all medical suggestions thoroughly. Any additional avenues you want to explore can be taken in addition to your doctor's advice.

Acupuncture: The combination of herbs and acupuncture can bring warmth to the reproductive system when blood congestion, or coldness, is responsible for amenorrhea. When it comes from stress-related sources (overexercise, the stress of sports competition, or birth control pills), acupuncture can support your system.

Chiropractic: Structural problems with your pelvis can affect the menstrual cycle. Spinal alignment helps the blood flow and nerve supply to your reproductive system without interference. In cases where structural imbalances are the cause for amenorrhea, chiropractic can be an effective solution.

THE CANDIDA ALBICANS DIET

Candida albicans is a yeast that lives peacefully in our intestinal tract, kept in check by intestinal bacteria. When its balance is upset, it can grow rapidly and cause a number of health problems.

Candida's growth can be stimulated by one or more of the following factors:

1. Repeated or long-term use of antibiotics, which kills off the intestinal bacteria that normally keep the *Candida* in balance.

2. Birth control pills and progesterone suppositories, which increase progesterone levels and cause vaginitis.

3. Repeated pregnancies, which change the hormone balance.

4. High intake of refined carbohydrates (often sugar), which feed the yeast.

5. Cortisone and other drugs, which suppress the immune system and prevent it from keeping the *Candida* in check.

When the yeast form grows out of proportion, it can cause a type of vaginitis. As *Candida* proliferates, it can also change from a yeast to a fungus, which can travel through the intestinal barrier and cause more severe symptoms. When it penetrates the intestines with its long, rootlike structures, it allows partially digested food particles into the bloodstream. The immune system identifies them as foreign invaders and leaps to the rescue with a variety of white blood cells that perform various functions. When the immune system's balance is upset, white blood cells may fail to respond to true foreign material such as viruses or may run rampant and destroy normal cells in error. This can cause allergic reactions and lower our immune system. At this point, *Candida* becomes a systemic problem. It is more difficult to identify and includes a wide variety of physical and emotional symptoms. It is also more difficult to control than when it is in yeast form.

When *Candida* is simply a vaginal yeast infection, the immune system may not be involved to a great extent. However, when symptoms increase and vary, suggesting that colonies of yeast may have been established in the body over a long period of time, a poor immune response is often present. In a weakened immune system, the invading fungus escapes destruction by white blood cells and continues to multiply in the tissues. One possible cause for persistent vaginal yeast infections is an immune system too weak to eradicate it. If you have a number of symptoms in addition to vaginal yeast infections, you may have an overgrowth of *Candida* in your body and a low immune response.

Orion Truss, M.D., author of *The Missing Diagnosis*, a book on *Candida*, has spent the last twenty years researching allergies and the immune system. He has found *Candida* symptoms to include:

abdominal discomfort	loss of libido (sex drive)
abdominal distention	loss of self-confidence
allergic reactions	menstrual cramps
anxiety	menstrual flooding and/or clots
constipation	migraine and sinus headaches
depression	rectal itching

diarrhea

esophagitis (inflammation of the esophagus)

irregular menstrual cycles

irritability

uncontrollable crying

vaginal discharge

vaginal itching

Presently, Dr. Truss believes *Candida* is best diagnosed through symptoms and response to treatment. A diagnosis would be further strengthened when the onset of symptoms correlates with one or more possible causes. If your depression, abdominal bloating, and constipation began after you took antibiotics, the probability that you have *Candida* increases.

Just as there is no simple diagnosis or test for *Candida*, there is no simple treatment. Stopping the growth of the fungus and driving it out of the tissues are the goals of a multilevel treatment that includes:

Immediate elimination of antibiotics, birth control pills, and other hormone-altering substances.

A diet designed to stop feeding the yeast.

Medical use of antifungal agents—such as Nystatin, or a homeopathic liquid, Candex—which permeate the intestines and help destroy Candida throughout the body.

Strengthening of the immune system through supplementation.

The diets required to starve out *Candida* eliminate all sources of yeast and fungus and all sugars and sweets, including lactose-containing dairy products, except for butter. Lactose is a form of sugar that feeds *Candida*. It is not easy for many people to avoid eating bread or using vinegar, which contains yeast, but it is the fastest way to eliminate the uncomfortable symptoms *Candida* brings. Gynecologists using this method remark that it is easy to induce women to follow it because they feel so miserable they will do anything to get better. I have found by adding supplements, the process is speeded up.

Mild cases of *Candida* (yeast infections and vague symptoms that are recent) will usually respond to the Candida Diet No. 1. Moderate *Candida* (chronic, severe yeast infections or definite, interfering symptoms), would best respond to the Candida Diet No. 2. Severe cases, which may have begun in early childhood or are debilitating (cannot work, difficulty functioning), would require the persistent efforts of the Candida Diet No. 3. Because of the complexities of this condition, I have slightly altered the format for these diets from others in this chapter, listing them separately from mild to severe, with recommended supplementations for each.

Nystatin, an antifungal available in tablet, pure powder, or suppository form from medical doctors and some women's clinics, speeds up this eradication. Candex, a liquid homeopathic preparation, contains a greatly diluted extract of *Candida*. It seems to lessen the immune response (the symptoms you feel) and helps produce antibodies to destroy the yeast throughout the body. The combination may be helpful in particularly stubborn cases, although I have found excellent results with diet, Candex, and supplements to help build the immune system. Both Candex and Nystatin may initially produce intensified reactions, but these are usually a sign of *Candida* flaring up before dying off. I see this as a positive sign, and advise women to adhere to their diets 100 percent at this time for fastest results.

Why the Candida Albicans Diets Work: Each diet is designed to stop feeding the yeast or fungus, reestablish helpful intestinal bacteria to keep future yeast from overproducing, and kill off existing colonies in the tissues. The suggested supplements help the immune system regenerate itself and provide future protection.

Specifics of the Candida Albicans Diets:

Candida Diet No. 1: Mild For persistent vaginal yeast infections with no other symptoms. This diet will help you get the *Candida* under control and prevent recurrent outbreaks.

Eliminate	Reduce	Emphasize
sugar in all forms, including honey, except occasional whole fresh fruit	whole grains and starchy vegetables until symptoms lessen	Eggs, fish, chicken, turkey, seafood, lamb, and veal
fungus, molds, and yeast in all forms, including vitamins and minerals:	fruit and diluted fruit juices, which may cause yeast to grow	vegetables except corn and potatoes
most B vitamins (unless label states otherwise)	nuts and seeds (small amounts)	vegetables that inhibit the growth of *Candida:* raw garlic, onions, cabbage, broccoli, turnip, kale
most breads and commercial baked goods	beans and other legumes (small amounts)	
all alcoholic beverages		
mushrooms		
vinegar and all foods containing vinegar, including salad dressing, sauerkraut, green olives, pickled vegetables, and relishes		
some crackers (read labels carefully)		
fermented products including soy sauce (tamari) and tofu		
dry roasted nuts		
barbecued potato chips		
most commercial soups		
apple cider and natural root beer		
white flour		
bacon and other pork, which often contain molds		

Supplements for Candida Diet No. 1: Take for one month after symptoms stop:

Yeast-free multi-vitamin/mineral

1000 milligrams vitamin C, two times a day

Lactobacilus acidophilus tablets to increase intestinal bacteria

Candida Diet No. 2: Moderate For chronic vaginal yeast infections, or additional symptoms which prevent you from feeling really good, begin with this diet. If Diet No. 1 did not clear up your symptoms, incorporate these suggestions into your program as well.

Eliminate	Reduce	Emphasize
same as Diet No. 1	same as Diet No. 1, except for some whole grains: brown rice, millet, buckwheat, cornmeal	same as Diet No. 1
wheat, oats, rye and barley, which contain gluten and can feed *Candida*		
fruit and diluted fruit juices, high in fructose (fruit sugar)	herb teas and spices, which may contain molds	

Supplements for Candida Diet No. 2:

Yeast-free multi-vitamin/mineral

1000 milligrams vitamin C, four times a day

Lactobacilus acidophilus in large quantities (Ultradophilus, Maxidophilus, Superdophilus, and so on, with approximately 2 billion organisms per gram) to help repopulate the intestines. Take ½ teaspoon morning and evening on an empty stomach.

2 teaspoons olive oil with 2 teaspoons oat bran, three times a day, to help keep fungus from crossing the intestinal barrier

100 micrograms selenium for immune system support

400 iu dry vitamin E for immune system support

20,000 iu beta carotene for immune system support

Digestive enzymes, with pancreatin, after meals and before bed, to help digest the food you eat as well as undigested food particles in the bloodstream

Candex to improve immune response and eliminate the fungus

Candida Diet No. 3: Severe Some women are debilitated by *Candida* and cannot function at work or can barely get through the day. If you were exposed to high levels of antibiotics as a child, or if you have had severe symptoms for more than four years, go directly to this diet. If your symptoms did not clear up with Diet No. 2, advance to this one until they diminish.

Supplements for Candida Diet No. 3:

Yeast-free multi-vitamin/mineral

Digestive enzymes with pancreatin after meals and before bed

Eliminate	Foods You Can Eat
same as Diets nos. 1 and 2	eggs, fish, chicken, turkey, seafood, lamb, or veal, sautéed in a little butter or safflower oil or baked with vegetables.
dried meat and smoked meat, fish, or poultry, including sausage, hot dogs, luncheon meats, smoked turkey, and smoked salmon	steamed, sautéed, or baked vegetables, especially onions, garlic, cabbage, broccoli, turnips, and kale. All vegetables are fine except potatoes and corn, which are high in carbohydrates.
nuts and seeds, which may contain mold	
all grains, except a little rice and millet	
herb teas and spices	sautéed vegetables with eggs on rice cakes, or a vegetable omelet.
	salads seasoned with safflower oil and a little fresh lemon juice.
	gazpacho, tomato-based fish chowder, vegetable soup, chicken or lamb stew.
	small quantities of rice and millet. A cold rice salad with steamed vegetables, seasoned with oil and lemon juice; sautéed rice with shrimp, chicken, and vegetables, or simply steamed vegetables with either grain are a few ideas that will work on this program. Rice cakes, found in some supermarkets and health food stores, can be used instead of bread.
	vegetable sticks with guacamole dip (avocado, fresh tomatoes, onions, lemon juice, and a little salt) for a snack.

1000 milligrams vitamin C an hour (up to 10 grams/day) for immune system

Acidophilus in large quantities (some brands, Ultradophilus, Maxidophilus, and so on have approximately 2 billion organisms per gram) to repopulate the intestinal bacteria. Take ½ teaspoon morning and evening on an empty stomach.

2 teaspoons olive oil with 2 teaspoons oat bran, three times a day, to help keep fungus from crossing the intestinal barrier

100 micrograms selenium three times a day, for immune system

400 iu dry vitamin E two times a day, for immune system

20,000 iu beta carotene, for immune system

Pau D'Arco tea (taheebo tea), an herb tea from South America, which kills fungus, one cup three times a day

Candex to improve immune response and eliminate the fungus

Nystatin in powder form, available through gynecologists and clinics

As soon as you are free from symptoms, begin reintroducing a few foods slowly. The last ones to add would be yeast, vinegar, and mushrooms. It may be necessary for you to stay on the Candida Albicans Diet for a number of months. Gynecologists report a year or more is not unusual, but I have found by combining supplements with diet, it is often possible to go back to the Anti-illness Diet more quickly. The more thoroughly you are able to stay on these diets, the faster you can eliminate excess *Candida*. However, it is better to be on a modified diet than on no diet at all. A few of my patients would rather eat sugar or have a glass of wine occasionally even though it may mean being on the diet for a longer period of time.

Auxiliary Treatment:

Gynecology: For a doctor who understands your desire to use nutrition along with medication, for a diagnosis of your condition, and to monitor your progress. A doctor can also provide you with a prescription for Nystatin, if you would like to use this antifungal medication.

Nutritionist, acupuncturist, nurse practitioner, medical doctor, or other health-care professional: To provide you with Candex, the homeopathic preparation I have used so successfully, and to monitor your progress. Candex is available in a number of strengths, each one designed for particular degrees of *Candida* overgrowth. For this reason it is only available through health-care professionals, who can select the appropriate dosage for you and monitor your progress. Candex is manufactured by Seroyal Brands, Inc. If you are interested in finding someone in your area who is familiar with its use, call their toll-free number: 1–800–533–1033.

Acupuncturist: To improve your immune response, eliminate bloating, increase energy, and improve your digestion.

Psychologist: To help you integrate your new eating patterns into a comfortable, workable lifestyle. As your symptoms decrease and are eliminated, it is often helpful to have someone assist you in seeing yourself as the healthy person you are.

THE CYST AND TUMOR DIET:
FIBROCYSTIC BREASTS AND UTERINE FIBROID TUMORS

Breast and uterine cysts and ovarian or uterine fibroid tumors are nonmalignant tissue masses. Except for uterine cysts, which are rare, these masses are common in women approaching menopause and occur most frequently in women between twenty and the mid-forties. A change in hormone activity seems to influence their growth, as evidenced by an increased incidence in women who have had children after age forty, but their exact cause is not known. Fibrocystic breasts are often most painful before menstruation, when cysts enlarge and breasts become tender. Diet seems to play an important factor in their presence and is often effective in reducing or eliminating them.

Breast Cysts and Breast Cancer. One out of eleven American women will get either malignant or benign breast disease, one reason for you to have regular breast exams. The small lumps that can be most easily treated cannot be felt through manual examination, one reason for a more thorough medical exam (see Auxiliary Treatment).

There is disagreement as to whether women with fibrocystic breast diseases are high risks for breast cancer. Some studies claim they are at a twofold to eightfold greater risk, but in the National Women's Health Network newsletter, Maryann Napoli indicates this association has been overrated. Dr. Saar Porrath of the Woman's Breast Center in Santa Monica, Calif., agrees that breast cysts do not normally become malignant. Still, the anticyst diet he and others recommend could also be considered an anticancer diet: low in fats, caffeine, salt, and sugar.

Women with diets high in meat and refined carbohydrates have more breast cysts, Napoli reports. It is here the similarity between noncancerous cysts and breast cancer begins. In articles published in both the *International Clinical Nutrition Review* and *Nutrition Report,* high-fat diets are implicated in breast cancer. A study conducted at the Oklahoma Medical Research Foundation revealed that tumors in lymph nodes increased with increased dietary fat intake. A high meat diet is also high in fats, although animal fats are not the only culprit. In fact, the fats that seem to cause the most problems are the fatty acids found in margarine and solid vegetable shortenings. A diet that contains a lot of milk (a major source of animal fats) is also associated with increased incidences of breast cancer.

Medical researchers Stephen Seely of the University of Manchester, England, and Dr. David Horrobin, in Nova Scotia, conducted a study of women in twenty countries and found a correlation between high sugar consumption and breast cancer mortality. To prevent both malignant and nonmalignant masses, you should be on a diet low in sugar. Since insulin is needed for the growth of breast tissue, excessive insulin—produced by eating quantities of sugar—may be responsible for malignant tissue growth, according to Dr. Seely.

Reduction or elimination of breast cysts is possible with oral vitamin E therapy and by severely restricting caffeine in all forms, including many prescription and nonprescription drugs (Anacin, APC tablets, ASA compound, Bromo Seltzer, Doan's pills, Dristan, Empirin Compound, No-Doz, Trigesic, Darvon, Fiorinal, Percodan, and others). In an article in the *Journal of the American Medical Association*, Robert S. London, M.D., director of reproductive endocrinology at Sinai Hospital in Baltimore, Md., advocates the use of vitamin E. "We found absolutely no side effects in terms of clinical derangements," he announced, "and it worked in a high percentage of patients. The other therapies are all more dangerous or have more side effects." Oil-based vitamin E capsules cause gastrointestinal upsets in some patients, one reason many doctors and nutritionists advocate using dry E tablets.

Another study, which examined caffeine restriction and reported in *The Journal of Reproductive Medicine,* found 88 percent of the women who reduced their caffeine intake had improvements in breast cysts. There was a dramatic reduction compared to those women who continued using coffee, tea, and other caffeine-containing substances such as over-the-counter medications and chocolate.

Uterine and Ovarian Tumors. These can grow large enough to affect the menstrual cycle and cause abdominal discomfort. Many doctors suggest hysterectomies, although these masses usually stop growing and reduce in size after menopause, when fewer hormones that stimulate their growth are produced. There is less information about uterine and ovarian tumors than about breast cysts, but clinical observation and conversations with gynecologists indicate that their growth can sometimes be stopped with dietary changes. These changes include reducing fats, sugars of all kinds (including fruit), and protein, and increasing whole grains. This method frequently eliminates the need for surgery. In my practice, I have found success with a number of women who avoided surgery by changing their diets.

Evelyn was forty-seven years old when I first saw her. She was told she had uterine fibroids two months before, and several doctors strongly recommended a hysterectomy, which she wanted to avoid if possible. Shortly after she came to see me, Evelyn began bleeding vaginally. At this point, most women would have agreed to surgery, but she was determined to find another answer. I referred her to a gynecologist, who was not convinced surgery was necessary. "She is close enough to menopause that if we can stop these cysts from growing, nature will shrink them in a few years," he said. "They won't be a problem then."

Evelyn drank between five and ten cups of coffee daily and ate large quantities of meat and dairy products. She loved desserts and bread and butter, which she ate whenever she was under stress. I changed her diet to include a lot of whole grains and legumes. She eliminated all caffeine, dairy products, and white flour, and her fibroids stopped growing. Her gynecologist decided to monitor her closely but not perform a hysterectomy. More than two years later, she admits she is not as strict with her diet as she was at first. She eats some dairy products occasionally, and white flour creeps in from time to time. Still, her meat consumption is down, her total fats are considerably less than before, and she no longer drinks coffee. Regular visits to her doctor reveal no need for surgery. Her fibroids have stabilized. This conservative approach was taken after a thorough gynecological examination that eliminated the possibility of a more serious condition, on advice of her doctor, and under his supervision.

Why the Cyst and Tumor Diet Works: It reduces fats, meat, and caffeine, contributing factors to cyst and tumor growth. It is low in all sugars and refined carbohydrates because of the link between increased insulin production and breast tissue growth, and it contains supplementary vitamin E, found capable of reducing and often eliminating breast cysts. Normally, I prefer natural to synthetic supplements. But since all oils need to be reduced, and wheat-germ-oil-based vitamin E can become rancid more quickly than dry E, I recommend a synthetic, dry vitamin E as the safest form for women who have cysts. Dry E has an additional advantage of being more easily assimilated than its oil-based counterpart, as seen in research conducted by Jeffrey Bland, Ph.D.

Specifics of the Cyst and Tumor Diet: Fruit should be limited to one or two pieces a day. To limit your intake of sugar, whole fruit, rather than fruit juice, is preferred. It is not necessary or advisable to be on a totally fat-free diet, but reduce all fats, saturated and unsaturated. If you have not eliminated coffee yet, you must. Even one cup a day is too much if you have cysts or tumors. Substitute steam-extracted decaffeinated coffee, and move on to coffee substitutes such as Postum and herb teas such as chamomile or mint. Don't drink any coffee, black tea, or eat chocolate, although carob is permitted as long as it's not heavily sweetened and you eat it in small amounts. Avoid any drug with caffeine by reading labels carefully and checking with your doctor or pharmacist.

Supplements:

400 iu synthetic dry vitamin E, two times a day

Eliminate	Reduce	Emphasize
coffee, black tea, chocolate, other sources of caffeine	honey	whole grains
refined carbohydrates	fruit	vegetables
margarine	meats	some chicken and fish
Crisco and other solid vegetable shortening	dairy products	
	oil	
	fruit juices	
bacon, sausage, pork, and other fatty meats		
chicken skin		

Auxiliary Treatment:

Medical: A thorough gynecological examination to determine your condition and to monitor it. Mammography, thermography, or other methods of breast examination every year or two by a doctor who specializes in early detection of breast disease can improve your chance of detecting a problem before it becomes serious. Work with someone who understands your desire to use good nutrition in an effort to eliminate fibroid tumors or cysts. It is wise to have a doctor monitor your progress. You may feel you don't need one because you are getting results; however, don't assume you know more than doctors about whether your fibroids or cysts are under control or your condition is serious. Leave this in the hands of an expert diagnostician.

THE HERPES DIET

Herpes simplex is painful, annoying, and occasionally embarrassing. It is caused by a virus that is often dormant but becomes active under stress. It is a common problem, affecting from 50 percent to 75 percent of adults. There are two types of Herpes simplex, I and II. Herpes simplex I shows up as fever blisters or cold sores, which appear in and around the mouth. Herpes simplex II is genital herpes, and produces sores on the vulva, cervix, and other sites below the waist. Most outbreaks of herpes are painful, but when they appear on the cervix they may not be felt. Usually, a Pap smear identifies its presence, which may otherwise go unnoticed. Both types are transmitted by person-to-person contact, frequently through sexual intercourse, kissing, and oral sex.

Herpes simplex appears as small, itchy red sores that form blisters filled with clear fluid. Viral germs are contained in this fluid, which spreads as the blisters break. A crust and scab then forms over the sores before they disappear. In addition to being itchy, herpes simplex is also painful. At its onset, in fact, a burning or stinging sensation may precede the first nodules. It is at this time that treatment should begin—before a massive outbreak and severe discomfort.

Medical science has not agreed upon any solutions to herpes simplex, but one amino acid, l-lysine, has been found to clear it up, while another, l-arginine, seems to encourage its activity. L-lysine increases the destruction of l-arginine, so the more l-lysine you take, the faster you remove one of the irritants. There are two ways to use l-lysine. One is to increase foods high in this amino acid while decreasing those high in l-arginine. Another is to take supplements of l-lysine during an outbreak or as a preventive measure.

For some people, it is necessary to take l-lysine supplements in addition to dietary changes, since their bodies may not be able to digest or absorb sufficient quantities. In tests conducted by dermatologists reported by Richard Passwater, Ph.D., a biochemist known for his research on cancer, aging, and heart disease, l-lysine was found to be effective in 96 percent of the patients tested.

At this time there is no known cure for herpes, but most of the time it is inactive and causes no problems. Outbreaks are frequently brought on by stress. Sunburn, menstruation, colds, fevers, emotional problems, or overwork can all turn this sleeping virus into a raging flare-up of painful blisters. Therefore, the best preventive measure you can take is stress reduction in any form.

In numerous patients who came to me with either herpes simplex I or II, outbreaks stopped as soon as they reduced stress in their lives. We began by reducing nutritional stress with the Anti-illness Diet and added supplements, like l-lysine, to help handle other stresses more easily. Stress alters the amounts of l-lysine and l-arginine in the body, which can directly affect the growth of the virus.

After changing their diet and adding supplemental support, I ask my patients to get regular exercise, have massages when possible, use biofeedback, or meditate or practice some form of relaxation. Solving problems that contribute to tension are also important, and psychological counseling can be a valuable adjunct that frequently shortens the time it takes to eliminate them.

Why the Herpes Diet Works: It reduces stress, cuts back on l-arginine foods, which promote the viruses, and increases l-lysine foods, which help eliminate herpes. Additionally, it provides supplemental support to help the body withstand many forms of stress while you work to reduce or eliminate them.

Specifics of the Herpes Diet: It is important for you to reduce all kinds of stress in your life, beginning with nutritional stress. The Anti-illness Diet will help you do this, so do your best to adhere to it. The additional foods and supplements listed here are specifically designed to eliminate herpes outbreaks quickly.

Eliminate	Reduce	Emphasize
l-arginine foods:		l-lysine foods:
chocolate		eggs
peanuts		brewer's yeast
nuts		fish
seeds		potatoes
beans		
peas		
untoasted grains		

Supplements:

Active Herpes I or II:

1000 milligrams l-lysine three times a day for five days, then 500 milligrams l-lysine three times a day for six months

1000 milligrams vitamin C four times a day

B complex to help reduce stress

80 milligrams raw adrenal gland tablets for stress

Inactive Herpes I or II:

After herpes is inactive, you may add small amounts of beans and peas to your diet and reduce your supplementation to the following:

500 milligrams l-lysine three times a day

1000 milligrams vitamin C two times a day

B complex

Auxiliary Treatment:

Gynecologist: Regular examinations will rule out herpes on the cervix. In pregnant women, herpes simplex II is dangerous. It can be passed on to your baby during delivery as it travels through an infected birth canal, and this can lead to permanent nerve damage, brain damage, or death. For this reason, cesarean sections are often necessary in women who have active herpes.

Meditation or relaxation techniques: Each morning and evening, spend fifteen minutes or more doing some form of meditation or relaxation exercise. There are many cassette tapes that can teach you how to relax, such as *Mastering Stress* (noted in the beginning of this chapter under a description of Auxiliary Treatment). Additional books on the subject you may want to explore include *The Relaxation Response*, by Herbert Benson, M.D., and *Minding Your Body*, by Norman Ford.

Biofeedback: This technique monitors your heart rate or skin temperature with electronic instruments. The equipment gives feedback through sounds or lights to help you become aware of sensitive responses to stress you might otherwise overlook. After you become sensitive to how you feel under stress and when it is reduced, you can use visualization or meditation techniques without the electronic feedback.

Psychological counseling: Either group therapy or one-to-one counseling can help you see how stress sabotages your health as well as open you up to alternatives you may not be seeing. While you are perfectly capable of solving your own problems, seeing them through the eyes of an objective expert can help you get unstuck. For a listing of herpes discussion groups and subscription information for *The Helper*, a quarterly publication with current information on herpes research, send a self-addressed stamped envelope to HRC, Box 100, Palo Alto, CA 94302.

Massage: Swedish and other types of massage are not luxuries for you, but one of the quickest ways to remove physical stress. A full-body massage once every week or two can help you unwind and handle your life more easily. Facial massage, neck and shoulder massage, or just having a friend rub your feet are excellent means of relaxation.

Exercise: An excellent way to reduce stress is through daily exercise. Keep it simple and light, like a brisk walk, stretching exercises, yoga, swimming, or an easy jog. Avoid strenuous exercise until your condition is inactive.

Acupuncture: It eliminates pain, and in acute conditions can relieve and eliminate sores and other symptoms. Acupuncture can also reduce stress, which contributes to herpes, and increase your body's immune response to combat the problem.

Water therapy: jacuzzis, hot tubs, and baths can all help to melt away your troubles. Add bath oil and relaxing music for a soothing bath before going to bed.

THE MENOPAUSE DIET

Menopause, the time in our lives when our menstrual cycle stops, can be an easy transition both physically and emotionally. To some women it means their sexually attractive years are almost over, while others look upon it as a time of increased sexual freedom.

The hormonal changes that occur during menopause cause a number of symptoms, including hot flashes, moodiness, vaginal itchiness and dryness, that can be disturbing if they are not understood. Muscles can lose their tone, producing flabbiness and wrinkles, and there can be weight gain as the body's need for energy changes. While estrogen replacement therapy is a frequent medical recommendation to prevent some of these symptoms, it has been associated with an increased risk for breast and uterine cancer. Nutrition provides a safe alternative with many of the same benefits and none of the risks.

During menstruation, the pituitary gland, located at the base of the brain, releases hormones that stimulate our ovaries to release an egg. The ovaries produce estrogen to thicken the uterus lining and prepare a soft place for the egg and progesterone to break down this lining and get rid of it when it is not used. The elimination of this lining is menstruation.

As we get older, our ovaries are less responsive to the pituitary hormones. They release fewer eggs, make less progesterone and estrogen, and, along with the uterus, begin to shrink. When our body stops making eggs altogether, we are infertile, but hormone production has not come to a halt. Estrogen, which we continue to need, is manufactured in smaller amounts in our ovaries, liver, and adrenal glands. The adrenals increase their estrogen production—as long as they're not too exhausted from years of stress. Sometimes menopause occurs too rapidly for the adrenal glands to adjust their estrogen output. Then you may have menopausal symptoms. These occur most frequently when your hormonal system is undergoing changes. Once a balance has been reached, they stop.

Hot flashes, sometimes followed by sweating, are believed to be caused by a sudden decrease of estrogen production by the ovaries. They generally disappear after a year or two, when the body has adjusted to a lower level of hormones. You may wake up at night, dripping with perspiration; hot flashes can also cause redness and drenching during the day at inconvenient times, but there is nothing dangerous or unusual about them. Fortunately, I have found a combination of vitamins E and C will usually stop these flashes and their accompanying symptoms. Since a lot of alcohol, caffeine, and large amounts of food can raise our body temperature, keep your meals small and your alcohol and caffeine intake down.

Moodiness and depression are often a sign you need more B vitamins, and this may be helped with by taking B-complex, which can also help the liver in its estrogen production.

Since hormonal imbalances are usually responsible for vaginal itching, you may find it is eliminated with the use of vitamins E and C. Both vaginal itchiness and dryness can be treated topically with oils and creams if you want to avoid the risk of estrogen.

Exercise will not only help tone your muscles, it will also help burn up more energy and keep your weight down. As we age, we need less food for fuel. What we don't eat, we often wear. To be able to eat more, and to firm up muscles that would otherwise tend to grow flabby due to hormonal changes, exercise more. Exercising also produces endorphins that can reduce or eliminate moodiness and depression.

Why the Menopause Diet Works: It takes nutritional stress off your body, giving your adrenal glands and liver an opportunity to manufacture needed estrogen. It adds the vitamins that have been shown to eliminate some menopausal symptoms and includes a multi-vitamin/mineral to give you trace elements possibly lacking from your diet. Menopausal symptoms are symptoms of imbalance. This diet helps restore your body to a balanced state.

Specifics of the Menopause Diet: There is no better foundation for this diet than the Anti-illness Diet. It is important to eliminate foods that can stress the liver (chemicals and fats) and adrenal glands (caffeine and sugar).

Eliminate	Reduce	Emphasize
sugar	butter	whole grains
animal fats	desserts	cold-pressed vegetable oils
caffeine	honey	legumes
chocolate	alcohol	nuts and seeds (chewed well)
refined foods		dark green leafy vegetables
		fish
		eggs
		organic liver

Supplements:

multi-vitamin/mineral, to support the nervous system, help eliminate moodiness and depression, and provide a complete complement of vitamins and minerals to help bring your body into balance

800 iu dry vitamin E, to stop hot flashes

400 iu dry vitamin E, after hot flashes have stopped

1000 milligrams vitamin C three times a day, to stop hot flashes

Auxiliary Treatment:

Exercise: Any exercise that is not overdone and that doesn't put too much stress on your body is good. Stretching, to keep you limber, a brisk walk or bicycle ride (stationary or outdoors), yoga, and swimming are some of the best. To keep your upper arms from getting flabby, use Nautilus machines or work out at home with small weights, which you can buy for less than $20 in a sporting goods store. *Beautiful Body Building*, by Deidre S. Laiken, is a book that can teach you simple weight training at home. It won't make you too muscular, just firm up some flab. *The Sports Doctor's Fitness Book for Women*, by John L. Marshall, M.D., with Heather Barbash, includes a well-illustrated section on "Fitness over Forty-Five."

Psychotherapy: For some women, this change of life is frightening or disturbing. Nurture yourself. Get the support of a therapist who can help you see yourself as a constantly changing woman. You may want to join, or start, a weekly support group with other menopausal women to talk about your experiences and find that you are not alone in this experience.

Acupuncture: To eliminate any residual symptoms and strengthen your adrenal glands and liver for optimal estrogen production.

Meditation or relaxation exercises: Any stress you take off your body will improve your adrenal glands. What's more important, it will make you feel calmer and more able to cope with this very natural, unfamiliar stage of your life.

THE MENSTRUAL CRAMPS DIET

Some women have both PMS and menstrual cramps, others have only cramps. For this reason, the Menstrual Cramps Diet is separate from the Premenstrual Syndrome Diet. Menstrual cramps, or dysmenorrhea, may be either primary or secondary. Primary cramps may be sharp, in waves, or a dull ache. They usually begin with, or just before, menstruation, and last a day or two. Some women are bedridden every month with menstrual cramps or take a lot of over-the-counter medication to alleviate them. Neither situation is necessary. When you understand the cause, you can correct cramps at their source, rather than treat the symptoms.

Primary cramps are caused by an excess of certain chemicals that regulate cell functions. These are called prostaglandins and are produced during ovulation and continue to be made until menstruation begins.

The particular prostaglandins responsible for primary menstrual cramps are PGE2 and PGF1 and PGF2, manufactured in our bodies from arachadonic acid, found in animal and cooking fats. Women with severe cramps have much higher levels of PGE2 than women without them.

There is another type of prostaglandin, however, which is helpful to our system: PGE1. It reduces inflammation, helps lower cholesterol levels, and relaxes smooth muscles like the uterus. If you have eliminated all fats from your diet in an effort to stay slim, you may be a candidate for menstrual cramps. By eliminating even vegetable oils in salad dressings, you could be causing a problem that otherwise would not exist.

To prevent cramping, your body needs to stop manufacturing so much PGE2, inhibit existing PGE2 and make more PGE1. The prostaglandin inhibitors currently on the market, aspirin and Midol (aspirin with a muscle relaxant and caffeine), block all kinds of prostaglandins, including the helpful ones.

A better solution would be to make more of the prostaglandin that is helpful to our system—PGE1—and to decrease animal fats of all kinds. PGE1 is manufactured from the essential fatty acids found in unheated or cold-pressed vegetable oils and in oil of evening primrose, a supplement found in health food stores and some pharmacies. You can inhibit production of PGE2 with vitamin E, which will also reduce inflammation and will increase the blood supply through the veins. You can also drink some herb teas that reduce menstrual cramps by relaxing the muscles.

Secondary cramps are an indication that another medical problem exists, like endometriosis, fibroid tumors, pelvic inflammatory disease (PID), or an irritation coming from an IUD. These cramps may feel the same as primary menstrual cramps; however, in some cases other symptoms accompany secondary dysmenorrhea, such as painful intercourse or painful bowel movements, which may signal endometriosis. A change in diet could still be helpful, but if you have menstrual cramps, have a gynecological examination to determine which type you have and what other approaches may help alleviate them.

Why the Menstrual Cramps Diet Works: It increases vegetable oils, which contain the essential fatty acids needed to make PGE1, and adds herb teas to reduce cramping while this change is taking place. Additionally, it decreases animal fats, which contain arachadonic acid, used to make PGE2 and PGF1 and PGF2.

Eliminate	Reduce	Emphasize
	animal fats: dairy products (including butter), meat	cold-pressed vegetable oils, especially safflower
		herb teas, especially ginger, mint, chamomile, crampbark, black cohosh, blue cohosh
	cooking fats: margarine, coconut oil, palm kernel oil	

Ideas for using vegetable oils are found in the Premenstrual Syndrome Diet for PMT-C.

Supplements: The supplements given include those that help in the manufacture of PGE1: magnesium, vitamin B_6, vitamin C, and niacinamide.

200 to 800 milligrams vitamin B_6

250 to 500 milligrams magnesium

Multi-vitamin/mineral

1000 milligrams vitamin C

2 tablespoons cold-pressed safflower oil or 4 to 8 capsules of evening primrose oil (Efamol brand)

Auxiliary Treatment:

Gynecologist: For an examination to diagnose your condition and to rule out secondary dysmenorrhea.

Chiropractic: To check for and correct structural misalignments that could affect the pelvis, uterus, and ovaries. These structural problems could reduce blood flow and nutrition from reaching the reproductive area.

Acupuncture: To eliminate severe cramps when they are occurring and to promote easy flowing of menstrual blood.

Exercise: Any kind—from tennis and jogging to stretching and yoga—will help keep your blood flowing and stretch your muscles and reduce spasms. However, the deep breathing and stretching that comes with yoga can help your body relax more completely, reducing cramping.

Massage: All massage, especially to the lower back, can relax tight muscles, which contribute to menstrual cramps.

Biofeedback: Through this technique you can increase the blood flow to the uterus and reduce spasms and pain.

THE OSTEOPOROSIS DIET

Our bones are not hollow sticks that prop up our body, but living structures filled with calcium-containing cells that go through cycles of breakdown and renewal. When breakdown exceeds buildup, osteoporosis occurs.

Osteoporosis is a loss of bone density that can be caused by heredity, malabsorption of calcium into the bones, a sedentary lifestyle, stress, and a number of nutritional factors, including heavy smoking, alcohol abuse, oral contraceptives, a high sugar consumption, high phosphorus diet, and magnesium deficiency. It can result in fractures from such minor occurrences as a mild fall or a jar to the body. Osteoporosis increases with age, affecting women more than men and usually manifesting itself after menopause. Small-boned Caucasian women are the highest risk group, but 90 percent of all women over 75 have osteoporosis. The time to prevent it is now, through proper diet and exercise.

While bones contain high amounts of calcium, a thorough exploration of nutrition and osteoporosis in *Clinical Nutrition* explains many of the difficulties in solving osteoporosis simply by increasing calcium in our diets or by taking high-calcium supplements. We are told to take calcium supplements or eat more dairy products, and most dairy products are high in saturated fats—which we do not need. Calcium supplements do not guarantee that the calcium we take will be absorbed into our bones. *Nutrition Reviews* reports, for example, that in X rays of people with osteoporosis who ate diets high in calcium as compared with those who ate little calcium, they could find no correlation between the amount of calcium intake and bone loss.

Calcium is not easily absorbed or utilized, and malabsorption can cause other problems, such as atherosclerosis and arthritis, without preventing brittle bones. The subject of osteoporosis is a highly controversial one today. Although evidence is mounting to support the belief that less calcium, rather than more, may be better, many medical doctors feel this new approach is premature.

You must make your own decision based on as much information as you can get. There may not be conclusive evidence in your lifetime, but significant medical research, including articles in medical journals on calcium absorption by doctors such as Guy Abraham, have changed the course of health for many women. Based on this literature and clinical evidence reported to me by medical doctors, I have incorporated this program into my own life and believe there is enough information available now for you to prevent, and even possibly reverse, osteoporosis to some degree. If you are interested in obtaining a copy of Dr. Abraham's article, "The Calcium Controversy," send a self-addressed, stamped envelope to: Calcium Controversy, Health Choice Enterprises, P.O. Box 2004, Redondo Beach, Calif. 90278.

Here are some arguments in support of the less calcium, more magnesium approach. It is not the amount of calcium we ingest but how much we absorb that affects bone density.

Hydrochloric acid, produced in the stomach, aids in calcium absorption by breaking down calcium there. As we age, our stomach becomes less efficient at HCl production. In addition to age, drinking liquids with meals, drinking colas, eating quickly, and not chewing well, all contribute to low HCl production.

After the calcium is broken down in the stomach, it is absorbed through the intestines into our blood, then into the soft tissues, and finally, into our bones. To get calcium into our bones, we need hormones manufactured by the thyroid and parathyroid glands to control calcium balance. When these hormones are present, we need the vitamin D found in fish and fish liver oils to utilize them. Fortunately, our bodies can manufacture this vitamin from sunlight if it isn't present in sufficient quantities in our diet, as long as we spend some time outdoors each day.

Then there's the delicate calcium-magnesium balance. Although we need twice as much calcium as magnesium in our bodies, most of us eat too much calcium. To restore our bodies to balance, we need more magnesium and less calcium. This is nothing to be concerned about, because when our total calcium intake decreases, we use a greater percentage of it than when our calcium intake is high—a fact noted in one of the most respected textbooks on nutrition, *Modern Nutrition in Health and Disease*, by Robert S. Goodhart and Maurice E. Shils. A low-calcium diet may actually help guard you against osteoporosis.

Too much calcium, on the other hand, blocks the absorption of magnesium. A recent article on magnesium in *Surgery* points out that unless magnesium is replaced first, calcium may collect in the soft tissues, resulting in arthritis. Rather than increasing calcium, we need to increase magnesium in our diet with, for example, whole grains. Studies reported in *The American Journal of Clinical Nutrition* indicate an increase in dietary magnesium raised both calcium and magnesium levels.

Just as certain nutrients increase calcium absorption, others decrease this absorption and contribute to osteoporosis. For example, an excess of phosphorus prevents our bodies from using calcium by causing more calcium to be excreted. Many of our processed foods, such as cheeses, soft drinks, and meats, are high in phosphorus. In fact, meat has more than twenty times as much phosphorus as calcium, which is why a diet high in meats increases your risk of brittle bones.

Caffeine and sugar are foods that contribute to osteoporosis. Caffeine causes the body to excrete almost twice as much calcium as normal in solid wastes, and sugar causes large amounts to be excreted in the urine. Smoking and heavy drinking both lower calcium levels as well and should be reduced. If you have the beginnings of osteoporosis, or are a high risk for this condition due to heredity, eliminate them completely.

Oxylalic acid (found in spinach, parsley, beet greens, chocolate, and bran) may be part of your calcium malabsorption problem; however, both magnesium and vitamin B_6, found in whole grains, counteract this problem. Oxylalic acid is an organic acid that combines with calcium to form an insoluble material that can lead to stones in the kidneys or gallbladder. It will not, however, prevent calcium eaten at the same time from being absorbed. There is no need to stop eating any of these vegetables. But chocolate, which also contains caffeine—the culprit cited above—and is high in fats does need to be eliminated. A high-fat diet, which prevents the absorption of many vitamins and minerals, is another contributor to calcium malabsorption.

Why the Osteoporosis Diet Works: It eliminates foods that cause calcium malabsorption or loss and emphasizes those containing both calcium and magnesium. Added to the Anti-illness Diet, it becomes an excellent preventive program. Current medical research will tell us some time in the future to what degree it can restore bone density where loss has already occurred. In the meantime, its possibilities for success and its common-sense indications can only improve your health.

In all the arguments surrounding osteoporosis, there seems to be universal agreement that a sedentary lifestyle and bed rest increase osteoporosis no matter how much calcium and other nutrients are taken, but that certain exercises prevent loss of bone density. These exercises work the weight-bearing bones of the legs, hips, and pelvis.

In a recent study of post-menopausal women aged sixty to sixty-nine, published in *Medicine and Science in Sport and Exercise*, bone density was measured in the most active women as compared with the least active. There was significantly less osteoporosis in the group of active women. Bone density in swimmers, however, was similar to those women who did not exercise. Although it is excellent exercise, swimming does not put any stress on the bones.

Eliminate	Reduce	Emphasize
caffeine	sugar in all forms	whole grains
processed meats and cheeses	fats	beets, peas, green peppers
soft drinks with phosphorus	protein intake	raw nuts, especially almonds
chocolate	dairy products	fish, especially haddock, flounder, cod, snapper
	nicotine	bananas, apples, nectarines
	alcohol	tofu

Supplements:

HCl if needed to absorb calcium in your stomach. Check with your doctor to determine your need for this, and refer to the Good Digestion Diet and the questionnaires in chapter 3 before taking any.

Multi-vitamin/mineral like Optivite, or

250 milligrams magnesium to help the intestines absorb calcium and magnesium

300 milligrams vitamin B_6 to help stop calcium malabsorption that occurs in high-oxylate foods such as spinach, parsley, and so on, unless your diet is high in whole grains

100 milligrams vitamin D supplement or, better still, a half-hour of sunshine a day

Auxiliary Treatment:

Exercise: The kinds of exercises that put stress on bones in your legs, as well as your hips and pelvis, include walking, jogging, bicycling (including stationary), hiking, and rowing. If you use Nautilus or other exercise equipment including free weights, you can exercise these bones as well.

Sunlight: For the manufacture of vitamin D. This is most easily obtained when you exercise. You do not have to be an athlete to take a brisk walk outdoors for fifteen to twenty minutes a day. More exercise is even better, but less may not be sufficient for the results you want.

THE PREGNANCY DIET

Pregnancy presents its own series of needs, including superior nutrition to both feed a growing fetus and support the mother. A growing fetus takes protein, vitamins, minerals—all the nutritional elements it needs—from our bodies. This can leave you depleted nutritionally. If you eat well but do not absorb some of your nutrients, they cannot be passed on to the fetus, and it in turn may be depleted. Experiments with pregnant animals have shown that when a nutrient is missing or low, deformities can occur throughout the fetus. The idea that a vitamin or mineral is needed for particular areas, like calcium for the bones, is a myth. We, and our developing babies, use all nutrients throughout our bodies.

The time to concentrate on becoming healthy enough to have a baby is *before* you become pregnant. Begin by adopting the Anti-illness Diet as your way of eating. It contains whole foods to build up your body and eliminates junk foods. Next, have a checkup complete with a blood panel to rule out any clinical abnormalities, indications that you are not completely well. If you have any minor problems, like indigestion (which could be a signal you are not using the nutrients from the foods you eat) or fatigue (which could mean you are run-down, anemic, or have a blood sugar imbalance), seek professional help to eliminate them now. These minor problems could affect your health and the health of your baby.

While you can "get away" with ingesting some substances when the only person you are feeding is yourself, they may have a detrimental effect on your baby. Alcohol, caffeine, and cigarettes have all been found to be harmful to fetuses. Because of biochemical individuality, we can only guess at how much is too much. You and your baby are better off without them. Reports in the *Journal of the Florida Medical Association* and the *International Clinical Nutrition Review* mention that alcohol in any amount during pregnancy could be damaging; smoking can prevent the fetus from absorbing nutrients and may result in significantly smaller babies. Jeffrey Bland points out that caffeine can cross the placenta and contribute to birth defects. If you want good health for yourself and your baby, and if you can possibly do it, stop drinking alcohol and caffeine and stop smoking.

You need an abundance of some nutrients when you are pregnant: protein, to build muscles and tissues in the fetus; vitamin B_6, to prevent edema and the nausea associated with morning sickness; iron, to manufacture more red blood cells for the fetus and placenta, and to guard against anemia in either of you; calcium, for the fetus's bone development; and zinc, which is taken from your diet rather than from your tissues. Good food alone will not supply you with all of these.

Oral contraceptives decrease the amount of folic acid in the mother. This is a vitamin associated with iron, a lack of which can lead to anemia or depression. If you have taken birth control pills in the past, folic acid supplementation may be wise.

Your need for protein increases during pregnancy, partially because it is a necessary nutrient for the growing fetus and also because more amino acids are excreted at this time. Still, be careful not to overload your system. Listen to what your body is telling you. The Anti-illness Diet, with some dairy products added, should provide you and your baby with all the protein the two of you require. Be sure to include eggs, nuts and seeds, beans, legumes, and both fish and chicken. You may want two small servings a day. If you can digest dairy products and develop a taste for milk during your pregnancy, by all means, drink some. If you have difficulty with lactose, a little yogurt might be the answer.

In *A Physician's Handbook on Orthomolecular Medicine,* John Ellis, M.D., who has received international recognition since 1961 for his research with vitamin B_6, reports eliminating edema in pregnant women with from 50 to 300 milligrams of B_6 a day. He has found a greater need for this vitamin in pregnant than nonpregnant women. Since consciously eating foods high in vitamin B_6 would only result in 5 milligrams a day, he suggests the need for supplementation.

We need enough iron to prevent anemia, for our baby's growing blood supply, and for the placenta. The fetus gets iron from its mother's body and from the foods she eats. Iron absorption, usually slow, is improved during the last two-thirds of pregnancy. Still, we need iron-rich foods, such as lean meat, organic liver, and dark green leafy vegetables, at this time—when our need for iron increases to about six times that of men's. Additional iron supplements in a high-quality multi/vitamin mineral should be sufficient.

Calcium needs are increased with pregnancy, but there are many research scientists and gynecologists who believe a normal diet that contains some dairy products is sufficient, especially since calcium absorption is increased at this time. With a whole-foods diet rich in calcium and magnesium, such as whole grains and legumes, little additional calcium supplementation should be required.

Zinc, often lacking in our diets, helps us absorb vitamins, especially B-complex. When sufficient quantities are lacking in animals, it produces cleft lip and cleft palate. High amounts of calcium prevent it from being absorbed, so if you increase calcium during pregnancy, zinc must be increased, as well. Since much of this trace mineral is found in fresh fruits and vegetables grown in rich soil, and much of our food is grown in mineral-depleted soil, zinc is a valuable element to add to your diet.

Why the Pregnancy Diet Works: It eliminates harmful substances that can deplete you and the fetus of necessary nutrients or interfere with their absorption and utilization. It concentrates on those nutrients that build healthy babies, while leaving you strong after you give birth. With proper nourishment, postpartum blues, often caused by insufficient vitamin B-complex, are unnecessary.

Specifics of the Pregnancy Diet: During pregnancy and for six months before, your diet should consist of the best quality foods you can find. You are "in training," preparing your body to receive an important gift that deserves, and needs, the very best nutrients. On such a diet, a weight gain of twenty to thirty pounds is often sufficient. Most literature suggests 75 grams of protein a day for pregnant women.

In addition to eating well, guard against harmful substances that could cause both of you unnecessary problems. Check with your doctor about the safety of any prescription medications you are taking and avoid all recreational drugs.

Eliminate	Reduce	Emphasize
alcohol	sugar	whole grains
cigarettes	refined foods	fresh fruits and vegetables, especially dark greens
caffeine		
foods with additives and preservatives		quality proteins, including lean meat, some dairy products, combined proteins and legumes
marijuana and other drugs		

Supplements:

Multi-vitamin/mineral

An additional 60 milligrams iron, if you have or suspect an iron deficiency

800 micrograms folic acid, unless included in the multi-vitamin/mineral

50 milligrams B_6 (pyridoxine) in the morning and at night. With edema, this amount may be increased to 150 milligrams; take twice a day, since any excess is excreted in the urine.

Auxiliary Treatment:

Gynecologist: To monitor your condition and advise you about nutritional changes as they are needed in various stages of pregnancy. Choose a doctor who understands and shares in your concern for good nutrition. They exist and are worth searching for.

Exercise: Your body needs flexibility, good muscle tone, and plenty of oxygen as it goes through some of the most dramatic changes it is likely to experience. If you already exercise, keep doing so at a rate that is comfortable. With the exception of heavy weight training, almost all exercise is beneficial. If you do not exercise, begin by walking half an hour a day. Stretching exercises and yoga can help you remain flexible and increase your oxygen intake.

Chiropractic: As your abdomen expands, more pressure is placed on your back to support it. When your spine is straight and your back muscles strong, you will have less of a tendency toward backaches. Chiropractic can help your body handle these new pressures by aligning your spinal column and strengthening weak muscles needed for support.

THE PREMENSTRUAL SYNDROME DIET

Premenstrual syndrome (PMS)—also called premenstrual tension (PMT) and premenstrual tension syndrome (PMTS)—consists of a wide variety of symptoms that begin from two weeks to several days before menstruation and subside or disappear when menstruation begins.

A survey of 2000 French women, reported in "Nutrition and the Premenstrual Tension Syndrome" in the *Journal of Applied Nutrition*, found that 74 percent believed PMS was part of menstruation. It is not. It can be eliminated, and it can be eliminated naturally. While some gynecologists advocate drugs such as progesterone for PMS, Dr. Guy Abraham believes in nutrition as "the safest, most efficient, and most acceptable form of therapy presently available."

Poor or unbalanced diets are often the cause of PMS, and good nutrition is a major part of the solution. PMS seems to be increasing as we seek out the richest ice cream, the most buttery croissants, and other rich foods high in fats and refined carbohydrates, which are causing mild to severe discomfort every month. We lunch on cottage cheese and yogurt to keep our weight down, unaware that too much calcium causes premenstrual anxiety and mood swings. Today's American diet has become PMS-promoting.

Stress also contributes to PMS. Many vitamins and minerals are critical to the prevention and elimination of PMS, but magnesium may head the list. It aids our body in absorbing calcium and vitamin B_6, both antistress factors. Stress blocks the absorption of magnesium itself and increases its excretion. Because our body does not know how to hold on to magnesium as it does with calcium, and because our diets high in dairy products and processed foods contain little magnesium, many of us are magnesium deficient. This depletion occurs in each subgroup of PMS and must be corrected through diet and supplementation before we can be completely free from monthly discomfort.

In a research study I conducted with Dr. Abraham studying the effects of nutrition and supplementation on women with all varieties of PMS, published in the *Journal of Applied Nutrition*, March, 1985, we found dietary and supplement changes resulted in a significant increase in both liver function and hormone production. At the same time, PMS symptoms were greatly decreased or completely alleviated. This study shows it is possible to eliminate the causes, as well as the symptoms, of PMS.

PMT-A (anxiety) is characterized by anxiety, mood swings, irritability, and nervous tension. These occur, in part, from high levels of estrogen and low levels of progesterone. Estrogen stimulates the central nervous system, which can lead to anxiety, while progesterone calms it down. While progesterone therapy may seem a likely answer, it addresses the symptom and not the cause, which several researchers believe is a deficiency of B_6 and magnesium. These factors are able to raise progesterone levels, and a high-fiber diet will increase excretion.

Dopamine is a chemical produced in the brain that balances out the effects of adrenalin and other chemicals that cause anxiety, irritability, and nervous tension. Magnesium deficiency results in less dopamine. B_6 is also thought to contribute to low dopamine levels. We need adequate amounts of both magnesium and B_6 to help raise dopamine. In addition, B_6 increases magnesium in cells, and in turn magnesium helps in the utilization of B_6 and other B vitamins.

Dairy products could be contributing to your PMT-A symptoms. They contain calcium with no magnesium. We have a continual need for magnesium-rich foods, such as whole grains, beans, and vegetables, since our bodies have not learned to store it. Instead, we eat foods made with white flour—which has no magnesium—avoid beans and other legumes because we believe they are fattening, and eat a lot of dairy products. In addition, the lactose in dairy products increases our excretion of magnesium, as does refined sugar.

To eliminate PMT-A, B_6 and magnesium supplements are often initially necessary, as is the elimination or reduction of foods high in calcium with little or no magnesium or high in refined sugar. Caffeine stimulates the central nervous system and may aggravate your symptoms. Exercise is good for everyone, but especially for women with PMT-A, and outdoor exercise seems to be particularly beneficial.

Specifics of the PMT-A Diet: The Anti-illness Diet is, to a great extent, an anti-PMS diet. It is important to follow it as completely as possible for all forms of PMS. In many instances where mild PMS symptoms are present, this diet alone may eliminate them. In other cases, following these specific dietary instructions along with supplementation will be necessary.

The key to this diet is to greatly reduce all dairy products and add foods high in calcium *and* magnesium. To break the craving for dairy products, which is a strong one in many people, I suggest you eliminate all dairy products temporarily. This will make it easier for you to break the old eating patterns that may have resulted in your PMS and will give you faster results. I have found this approach particularly successful with my patients, who lose excess weight as well as their PMS when they stop eating dairy products. After their symptoms are gone, they are surprised how little they care about a food group they once craved. At that point, small amounts of dairy products added to a good diet will usually not result in any recurrence of PMT symptoms.

Eliminate	Reduce	Emphasize
all dairy products except butter		whole grains
refined sugar		legumes
caffeine: coffee, black tea, chocolate, maté tea, guarana		dark green vegetables
		all vegetables, for fiber

Supplements for PMT-A:

Multi-vitamin/mineral (Optivite), 3 tablets twice a day after breakfast and lunch, or

250 to 500 milligrams magnesium

300 to 600 milligrams B_6 (pyridoxine)

Auxiliary Treatment for PMT-A:

Gynecology: A doctor who understands a dietary approach can be a valuable ally in monitoring your progress. He or she can also adjust your supplements if your PMS is so severe it does not respond to the dosages suggested. In my practice I have worked successfully with hundreds of women with premenstrual syndrome. When symptoms are severe, higher doses of vitamins and minerals bring much faster results; however, it is best to get specific information for your body from someone familiar with this approach. You can get additional information on doctors, nurses, nutritionists, and clinics familiar with the use of diet and supplementation from the following:

Health Choice Enterprises (Patrice Dowling)
P.O. Box 2004
Redondo Beach, CA 90278
(213) 379–7700

Health Options (Marilyn Seach-Koll)
P.O. Box 1917
Aptos, CA 95003
(408) 662–3544

Madison Pharmacy (Marla Ahlguinn and Dave Meyers)
1603 Monroe St.
Madison, WI 53715
(800) 558–7046 (this is a toll-free number)

Optimed of Georgia (Maurice Hider)
552 Old Mill Court
Norcross, GA 30093
(404) 873–9013

Psychotherapy: It is emotionally stressful to suddenly be free from physical and mental discomforts. You are now responsible for your actions. You are no longer being driven by biochemical imbalances. Now you are ready to discover who you really are and how you feel when you feel well. This can be disorienting for someone who is used to being manipulated physically and emotionally every month by her biochemistry. A therapist can help you make this transition as you begin to establish new patterns in your life.

Stress-reducing techniques: Relaxation techniques, meditation, yoga, stretching exercises, biofeedback, massage.

Exercise: At the minimum, a twenty-minute walk, three times a week. At best, four to six days a week of exercise to reduce stress and keep your body healthy. If you participate in outdoor sports or are willing to exercise more, you will probably get even greater results.

Acupuncture: To help tone your entire body and concentrate on energizing your reproductive system.

PMT-H (hyperhydration) is characterized by edema, including premenstrual weight gain of from one to three pounds, abdominal bloating and tenderness, tender breasts (sometimes with cysts), and swollen hands and feet. Water retention can come from too much salt or too much sugar. Diuretics are often given to eliminate excess water, but they only address the symptom, not the cause, and make the condition worse.

Salt retention, resulting in water retention, can be caused by too much aldosterone, a hormone produced by the adrenal glands. This hormone is often elevated before menses in women with PMT-H. This excess aldosterone can come from too much physical or emotional stress, a magnesium deficiency, too much estrogen, or too little dopamine. Besides being caused by a magnesium deficiency, aldosterone itself increases the excretion of magnesium in the urine. Diuretics cause more of a magnesium deficiency, and the symptoms of this subgroup are likely to worsen after diuretics have been used over a period of time. Taking magnesium is the only way to break this cycle, along with taking B_6, which supresses the production of aldosterone and results in less water retention. Excess estrogen is eliminated in a high-fiber diet, and dopamine is increased with B_6 and magnesium.

Most of us don't think of sugar as causing water retention, but it can. Our kidneys excrete excess water and salt with the help of ketoacids, which are formed when we eat very little sugar and have a low insulin output. Eating sugar increases insulin, supresses ketoacids, and causes the kidneys to hold on to water and sodium.

Specifics of the PMT-H Diet: The nutritional answers to this form of PMS are simple: keep salt and sugar intake to a minimum. Less stress will also contribute to getting free from symptoms, as will supporting your diet by emphasizing foods high in B vitamins.

Eliminate	Reduce	Emphasize
refined sugar	fruits	whole grains
fruit juices	salt	eggs
		fish
		nuts and seeds
		brewer's yeast
		organic liver

Supplements for PMT-H:

Multi-vitamin/mineral (Optivite), 3 tablets twice a day after breakfast and lunch, or

250 to 500 milligrams magnesium

300 to 600 milligrams B_6 (pyridoxine)

Auxiliary Treatment for PMT-H:

See auxiliary treatment for PMT-A, especially acupuncture to help reduce water retention quickly, gynecology, and psychotherapy.

PMT-C (craving) is characterized by a craving for sweets (often chocolate) and an increased appetite for carbohydrates. When large amounts of sugar are eaten, headaches, fatigue, heart palpitations, or fainting may follow. Often, an uncontrollable sugar craving accompanies stress. These hypoglycemia symptoms are a result of increased insulin secretion, which comes from a need for magnesium and essential fatty acids. Too much salt can also trigger this craving, since table salt enhances the absorption of sugar in the intestines.

In some women, the only food that will satisfy their sugar craving is chocolate. The need for magnesium can be seen more clearly here, since chocolate is extremely high in magnesium. When your magnesium balance is restored, chocolate cravings miraculously disappear.

In addition to more magnesium, PGE1, one of the hormonelike substances called prostaglandins, is necessary to break the pattern of this type of PMS. Prostaglandins are made from the chemicals we ingest in fatty acids, sources for which are meat, dairy products, nuts, seeds, and vegetable oils. PGE1 is a prostaglandin made from the *essential fatty acids* (EFAs), found in cold-pressed vegetable oils, and vitamins and minerals such as vitamin C, B_6, niacinamide, zinc, and magnesium. Heat destroys the EFAs required to make PGE1. Other inhibitors include animal fats, margarine, alcohol, and stress.

To eliminate this form of PMS, increase your complex carbohydrates (particularly whole grains and legumes); stop eating refined sugar and drinking alcohol if possible and reduce them to a minimum if not; limit your salt intake; and reduce all animal fats, cooked vegetable oils, and margarine. To help your body manufacture PGE1, add two tablespoons of cold-pressed safflower oil to your diet. Use it in salad dressings, over steamed vegetables instead of butter, and add it to cold pasta salads or tabbouli. You can also add it to tomato juice with a little lemon for a morning drink or put in in your breakfast protein drink. A simpler but more expensive solution is to take oil of evening primrose capsules, found in health food stores. Additional magnesium supplements are beneficial in helping keep hypoglycemic-like symptoms from occurring.

Specifics of the PMT-C Diet: The key to this diet is to reduce animal fats, sugar, and salt, and to increase cold-pressed vegetable oils and complex carbohydrates.

Eliminate	Reduce	Emphasize
refined sugar	fruits	whole grains and legumes
fruit juice	salt	cold-pressed vegetable oils, especially safflower
	animal fats	

Supplements for PMT-C:

300 to 600 milligrams magnesium

2 tablespoons cold-pressed safflower oil each day, or

1000 milligrams primrose oil (Efamol brand) twice a day, beginning three days before symptoms are due and taken until menstruation begins

½ teaspoon brewer's yeast, increasing dose gradually to 2 tablespoons

1500 milligrams of 1-glutamine powder (an amino acid) sprinkled over fresh fruit or added to diluted fruit juice as needed, to eliminate sugar cravings, if all else fails

Auxiliary Treatment for PMT-C:

See auxiliary treatment for PMT-A, especially gynecology, psychotherapy, and acupuncture.

PMT-D (depression) is characterized by depression, forgetfulness, crying, confusion, and insomnia. It can include difficulty verbalizing and lethargy. Some women become suicidal. It is almost always accompanied by PMT-A. When it is not, Dr. Abraham recommends psychotherapy in addition to dietary changes and supplementation.

Premenstrual depression can come from a number of factors. One is a need for tyrosine, an amino acid. Another is increased stress, which accompanies hormonal changes and which causes the adrenal glands to secrete a depressant to the central nervous system. B vitamins and magnesium support the adrenal glands but are often deficient in conditions of stress. The B vitamins also contribute to a reduction of depression by helping the brain produce antidepressant chemicals.

Premenstrual depression may also be a result of lead absorption and retention. We are exposed to lead in the air, water, and foods we eat. For protection against lead, we need magnesium. It normally keeps the intestines from absorbing lead, helps move it out of the bones, and increases its excretion. Excessive progesterone may also cause depression, and since progesterone is an option some women may consider to eliminate premenstrual syndrome, you should know it has the potential of making your PMT-D worse if your progesterone level is already normal.

This subgroup of PMS can be helped with magnesium-rich foods and supplementation, especially when lead toxicity may be present. Hair analysis is one method of determining lead toxicity, but since extra magnesium is often needed to eliminate other premenstrual symptoms, you may decide to increase this mineral rather than getting a hair analysis. Tyrosine, an amino acid found in health food stores, can increase mental alertness, and B vitamins can help reduce stress. Meditation, yoga, or relaxation exercises are also useful in stress reduction.

Specifics of the PMT-D Diet: Use the same dietary guidelines as with PMT-A.

Supplements for PMT-D:

Multi-vitamin/mineral (Optivite), 3 tablets twice a day after breakfast and lunch, or

250 to 500 milligrams magnesium

300 to 600 milligrams B_6 (pyridoxine)

3 to 6 grams 1-tyrosine (half in morning, half at noon) for depression, if needed

Auxiliary Treatment for PMT-D:

See auxiliary treatment for PMT-A, especially psychotherapy, gynecology, stress-reduction techniques, and exercise.

THE STRENUOUS EXERCISER'S DIET

Today more women than ever before are running marathons, completing triathlons, and entering bodybuilding competitions. Vigorous exercise has become daily routine for thousands of other women who will never participate in these sports, whose goals are to feel more fit, have more energy, tone their muscles, lose weight, shape their bodies, or feel stronger and more powerful. This diet is designed for all women who train long, hard hours five or more times a week. If you run, take an aerobics class, bicycle, lift weights, use Nautilus equipment, or play tennis or racquetball and consistently push your body, you have different nutritional needs than less active women.

Contrary to popular belief, exercising does not mean you need more protein. In fact, a high-protein diet may be counterproductive to a heavy workout. It can result in digestive problems, overworked kidneys, overheating, and the potential for becoming dehydrated. Your best source of energy is unrefined carbohydrates, such as whole grains, legumes, and starchy vegetables. They are best for anaerobic (stop and start) exercise, like sprinting, tennis, and racquetball; they supply needed fuel for aerobic endurance training (running, swimming, biking); and they are digested rapidly, making them more available for immediate use. According to Robert S. Goodhart and Maurice E. Shils in *Modern Nutrition in Health and Disease*, your body uses fats when you're resting but needs carbohydrates during both moderate and heavy exercise. At least 60 percent of your diet should be complex carbohydrates.

You need enough carbohydrates to replace sugar (glucose) that has been used up and enough protein to repair muscles broken down during exercise. Excellent results in repairing muscles have also been reported with a new, but proven substance—amino acids. A diet high in carbohydrates supplies both your brain and muscles with necessary glucose, but small amounts of dietary protein are sufficient for most athletes.

In addition to carbohydrates to replace glucose, the B vitamins found in whole grains help the body *use* glucose. These vitamins are also found in brewer's yeast and raw nuts and seeds. Vitamin E, also contained in nuts and seeds, was reported in the *American Journal of Physiology* to increase the performance in athletes over those who did not take additional supplementation. Used to build new muscle tissues and improve the transportation of oxygen throughout the body, this important vitamin is also found in the cold-pressed vegetable oils recommended for other women's health problems (see the Premenstrual Syndrome Diet and the Menstrual Cramps Diet).

Vitamin C is helpful whenever you are under stress, and vigorous exercise is stressful. It is found in many fruits and vegetables, like broccoli, brussel sprouts, cabbage, cauliflower, collard and turnip greens, kale, lemons, oranges, papayas, spinach, strawberries, and sweet peppers. Include some of these in your diet each day. The amount added to a multiple vitamin will provide any needed insurance.

Perhaps the two most important supplements needed by female athletes are iron and water. During a five-year study at the University of Hawaii, Ralph W. Hale, M.D., chairman of the department of obstetrics and gynecology, reported women athletes felt and performed better when their iron level was higher than the clinical standards for blood tests. Organic liver (sold in some health food stores), oysters, and dark green leafy vegetables are all high in iron. Include at least some on a regular basis. Dr. Jackie Puhl, a sports physiologist with the U.S. Olympic Committee, reports in *Nutrition Action* that performance may be adversely affected even before signs of clinical anemia. If you have an IUD and are menstruating heavily, you may have low iron. It is not advisable, however, to take high amounts of iron supplements unless you are certain your iron level is low. Too much iron can be harmful to you and has been of growing concern to the medical community. It can lead to underfunctioning of the endocrine glands and cardiac problems. The amount of iron in most multi-vitamin/minerals is usually sufficient to meet the needs of even very active women. Take additional iron supplements only if laboratory tests indicate you have a deficiency.

Keeping your body supplied with plenty of water is a challenge for the athletic woman, since thirst is not an accurate indication of how much you need. Water makes up 53 percent of your body weight and is lost through sweat during exercise. In addition to being necessary for circulation and the elimination of liquid wastes, it helps regulate your body temperature. Plain water is absorbed more quickly than liquids containing small amounts of sugar. Because your performance can be affected by a rapid loss of even a small percent of your body weight, drink some water before and during exercise when it will not interfere with your activities. Replenish your water supplies completely by weighing yourself before and after exercise. The weight you lose is water needed for your health and best performance.

High-quality amino acids taken after a workout help rebuild muscles quickly and effectively. Muscles need protein to rebuild, and amino acids are the fastest way to bring these building blocks into the muscles broken down by strenuous weight-training or running workouts. Safer than steroids and 80 percent as effective, specific amino acid formulas have been used the past few years by world-class athletes and bodybuilders to improve performance, prevent tissue wasting, and hasten recovery time.

An article in the *American Journal of Sports Medicine* reports that the irreversible side effects of steroids on women include a deepening voice, facial hair growth, baldness, and an enlarged clitoris. Other side effects (irregular menses, smaller breasts, uterine atrophy, and fluid retention) may reverse after steroids have been stopped. Unlike steroids, amino acids have no adverse side effects when taken in a balanced formula along with a multi-vitamin/mineral that supplies needed nutrients to help your body utilize the amino acids.

Athletes I have counseled who are taking an amino acid formula find enhanced performance, more definition in bodybuilding, and no sore muscles no matter how strenuous their workout. The formula I use is a pharmaceutical grade (the highest grade) amino acid combination called Aminoform, distributed internationally in health food stores by Integrated Health, Inc. This formula has been designed for body shaping and to avoid loss of muscle tissue during fasting or severe weight-loss programs. Many world-class bodybuilders are now using this same formula with great success. It can also be taken after any strenuous exercise routine, including endurance sports.

Another amino acid combination, Aminolete, is designed to produce enhanced performance during such endurance sports as swimming, running, and biking. At present, Aminolete is only distributed through doctors and health-care professionals by Tyson & Associates, parent company to Integrated Health. For more information, write them at 1661 Lincoln Blvd., Suite 300, Santa Monica, CA 90404.

Much has been said about the use of singular amino acids such as ornithine and arginine. Unfortunately, large amounts of these two amino acids can contribute to giantism—enlarged bones. When bones grow larger after maturity, they do not contain more calcium, and whatever other minerals they contain as well must be spread more thinly over a larger area, resulting in an increased possibility of osteoporosis. Because taking large amounts of individual amino acids may cause imbalances, I don't advise taking an incomplete formula, and always accompany a balanced compound with a multi-vitamin/mineral to supply the additional nutrients necessary for complete amino acid assimilation.

A word to the woman who exercises for weight loss: don't waste your time trying to spot reduce with specific exercises. All exercise stimulates the release of fats from fatty deposits, and you'll lose fat from the area where most is concentrated. If your thighs are where you hold most of your excess fat, a long daily walk will get them thinner even faster than doing thigh exercises a few dozen times.

Why the Strenuous Exerciser's Diet Works: It provides you with the complex carbohydrates needed for muscle energy and the nutrients that best support heavy exercise. It reduces your fat content to help you concentrate on better muscle performance and more definition where desired, and it eliminates foods that do not contribute to your mental and physical performance.

Specifics of the Strenuous Exerciser's Diet: Don't concern yourself about getting enough protein, even if you're a vegetarian. This diet is high in complex carbohydrates: whole grains, legumes, and nuts and seeds. When two or more of these are combined during the day, they form complete proteins. Athletes who are complete vegetarians get their necessary protein through combining these foods. One helping of high-quality, low-fat protein, such as a skinned chicken breast, a few slices of turkey, four ounces of broiled fish, or a little tofu added to grains and vegetables is sufficient for most athletes. If you are looking for a more detailed dietary plan, you may want to read *The Complete Diet Guide for Runners and Other Athletes*, edited by Hal Higdon.

Eliminate	Reduce	Emphasize
refined foods	fats (including dairy products)	whole grains
caffeine		starchy vegetables
salt		legumes
dried fruit		iron-rich foods (organic liver, oysters, dark green vegetables)

Supplements: Begin taking small doses of amino acids, to allow your body to adjust to them. They are a very concentrated food. Start with one capsule a day, and increase gradually until you have reached the suggested dosage.

Multi-vitamin/mineral

3 Aminoform capsules upon rising with 6 to 8 ounces of water or diluted juice (wait ½ hour before eating), and 3 after any workout, with water or juice

2 to 4 capsules Aminolete, twenty minutes before endurance sport workout, taken with 6 to 8 ounces of water or juice on an empty stomach

400 iu dry vitamin E

Auxiliary Treatment:

Chiropractic: For alignment of bones and muscles for enhanced performance. Helps the body recover more quickly from major and minor sports injuries. Find a chiropractor who specializes in sports medicine or one who understands your desire for strenuous workouts.

Meditation and relaxation: A competitive woman bodybuilder taught me that vigorous exercise is as much in the mind as in the body. Learning how to focus your attention in the moment on the muscles you are using, and setting goals are important aspects of your training. The best athletes in all fields use visualization techniques to see themselves performing before the actual event takes place. Spend enough time learning how to use your mind to assist your body.

DIETS FOR THE CONTEMPORARY WOMAN: MINIMIZING THE DAMAGE

I have a sign on my office wall that says, FORGET PERFECTION. AIM FOR EXCELLENCE. It's not for my patients—it's a reminder to me that I'm not perfect and don't have to try to be more than what I am at any given moment. Being imperfect is being human, and you may be one of those women who reflects her imperfection in her diet and health habits. Although you may know alcohol and oral contraceptives deplete you of certain nutrients, you may still choose to use them. Instead of berating yourself, admit it and do what you can to improve your health. If you're not ready to give up some of your habits just yet, the following diets take the "better than" approach. They may not represent perfection, but they can make a noticeable difference in how you look and feel.

THE BIRTH CONTROL PILL DIET

Although most methods of birth control have side effects and there is no perfect answer, for many women the benefits of taking oral contraceptives far outweigh any problems they may cause. If you are concerned about its side effects, an article in *The Lancet* indicated the best way to minimize them is to reduce the amount of estrogen or progesterone they contain. Check with your doctor to see if you are using one of the lower dosage brands.

Birth control pills result in specific vitamin and mineral deficiencies that you need to be aware of in order to correct.

Specific Nutrients Needed for the Birth Control Pill Diet: B_6 is depleted by using the Pill. This can result in premenstrual depression, nausea, water retention, and menstrual changes. In addition to eating whole grains, high in this vitamin, extra supplementation is often helpful. One good source is brewer's yeast.

B_{12} is also depleted by the Pill, a condition that can lead to anemia. Since this vitamin is particularly difficult to absorb, I suggest women on oral contraceptives use a high-quality vitamin formula, such as the one suggested in the beginning of this chapter. I have seen follow-up blood tests on women who used the Optivite formula that indicated absorption took place, while similar formulas did not produce such effective results. In addition to vitamins, you can supplement your diet with organic liver, lean meat, and fish, all containing B_{12}. Vegetarians must take supplements, since B_{12} is not found in sufficient quantities in meat-free diets.

A deficiency in biotin, another B vitamin, may result from taking the Pill. Symptoms are depression, fatigue, eczema, hair loss, and dry hair. The foods that contain good quantities of biotin include brewer's yeast, egg yolks, organic liver, and brown rice.

Folic acid is depleted by oral contraceptives and can contribute to anemia. It is needed for normal pregnancies in women who stop taking the Pill and then become pregnant. An article in the *International Clinical Nutrition Review* states folic acid should be replaced before pregnancy to prevent problems in the fetus. Since green leafy vegetables, liver, and brewer's yeast all contain large amounts of folic acid, they can be incorporated into your diet at all times to minimize the damage.

Vitamin C is lower in women who use oral contraceptives. Found in citrus fruits, garden peppers (both red and green), and most fruits and vegetables, it can be easily replenished through diet. Since you may want to protect yourself from infections and support your immune system, additional vitamin C may be taken during the day in supplements.

Vitamin E helps prevent blood clots by blocking the production of fibrin, a substance that helps clotting. When you have more estrogen than your body needs, which can occur when you take the Pill, you may be more prone to forming blood clots. Additional vitamin E helps keep estrogen levels normal. It is found in raw nuts and seeds and vegetable oils. If you are using cold-pressed safflower oil, you are getting a good source of vitamin E in your diet.

Zinc is depleted by the Pill, and it is found in whole grains and green leafy vegetables if they have been grown in zinc-rich soil. Despite the assertions of agriculturists, some of our food is not grown in soil enriched with minerals. If you are concerned about getting enough zinc (which also contributes to good skin and healthy adrenal glands—your stress center), you may want to take a supplement with added zinc. Foods high in this mineral include pumpkin seeds and, once more, brewer's yeast.

One benefit of oral contraceptives is increased calcium absorption. For this reason, you will most likely get enough calcium from such foods as whole grains, salmon, broccoli, and tofu (soy bean curd). There is usually no need to take additional calcium supplementation.

Suggested Dietary Changes for the Birth Control Pill Diet: The Anti-illness Diet is the foundation for this program, with the additions suggested in the preceding material.

Supplements:

Optivite or another high-quality multi-vitamin/mineral formula designed for women. The extra B_6 in these formulas is especially helpful for women on the Pill, and they both contain enough B_{12}, folic acid, biotin, and C to reverse and prevent further depletion.

1 to 2 tablespoons brewer's yeast. Begin with small amounts (¼ teaspoon) to avoid gas, and work up gradually to 2 tablespoons a day. Get in the habit of sprinkling it over your cereal or salads each day or mix it in breakfast drinks. If you have vaginal yeast infections or any other indication of *Candida albicans,* brewer's yeast is not advisable (see the Candida Albicans Diet).

THE CAFFEINE USER'S DIET

People drink coffee, tea, and cola drinks for their effect, their taste, or both. The stimulating and consequently harmful effects of caffeine on the adrenal glands has been discussed in more detail in chapter 4. Basically, caffeine stimulates the central nervous system, brain, and heart to give false energy and alertness you may have come to depend upon, elevates cholesterol levels, causes abnormally high or low blood sugar levels, and can cause gastric ulcers by irritating the stomach. Caffeine is associated with breast cysts (see the Cyst and Tumor Diet) and affects the fetus in pregnant women (see the Pregnancy Diet). It impairs the absorption of iron when drunk during or shortly after a meal, and it increases stress. To break this artificially induced condition and restore yourself to a more dependable energy, start cutting down on the amount you drink. Reduce your intake to the smallest quantity you feel comfortable with. If you feel deprived, you are likely to go back to your old habits.

A doctor once sent me a patient whose daily consumption of thirty cups of coffee was interfering with his health. During my own coffee-drinking heyday, I had consumed fifteen cups a day and remembered suffering from an acid stomach, digestive problems, and nervousness that I attributed at the time to my being energetic. Thirty cups was almost incomprehensible to me. Since I had no idea how much coffee it was reasonable to ask him to eliminate, I asked him.

He quickly replied that he could cut back to six cups a day. Within a week he had eliminated 168 cups of coffee—over 400 cups a month. Left to my own devices I would have suggested he reduce his intake more gradually, but he knew himself best. A month after we began working together, he was drinking only two cups a day. This is a dramatic example of the better-than approach.

Suggested Dietary Changes for the Caffeine User's Diet: The most important key to this diet is that less caffeine is always better. Use the following techniques to decrease the amount of caffeine in your diet:

1. Don't drink caffeine automatically. Think about whether or not you really want the coffee, tea, or cola before ordering it. If you don't want it, have something else.

2. Refuse refills. It's easy to drink from two to four cups of coffee or tea with a meal when it's being poured, for free, for you. Enjoy one cup without having an excessive amount.

3. Substitute a smaller cup for your large coffee mug. Psychologically you can drink the same number of cups and still physically reduce your intake.

4. Substitute other non-caffeinated beverages. Decaffeinated coffee and tea (water-processed whenever possible) and non-caffeinated soft drinks are preferable to those with caffeine. Add one-half decaf to each cup of coffee and gradually switch over to decaf. Include beverages without caffeine in your diet so you have other alternatives.

Suggested Dietary Changes for the Caffeine User's Diet: The Anti-illness Diet removes stimulating substances like caffeine and sugar and replaces them with energizing food, such as whole grains. As you incorporate this basic diet into your life, you will find less of a need for stimulants. When you feel a little tired in the afternoon, eat a piece of fruit instead of drinking a cola or a cup of coffee. Use food, not drugs, for energy.

Supplements:

B vitamins are antistress vitamins, and caffeine produces more stress. One B-complex formula taken morning and noon after meals can help reduce this stress.

80 milligrams whole raw adrenal tissue, found in health food stores, to reduce the initial fatigue that results from a reduction of caffeine stimulation. Take one tablet morning and noon after meals.

THE SOCIAL DRINKER'S DIET

In spite of some of the effects alcohol has on one's health (see chapter 4), some people still choose to drink it occasionally—and others on a more regular basis—without being alcoholics. A glass of wine with dinner or an occasional drink or two with friends will not result in cirrhosis of the liver, but some damage may still be occurring. You can minimize this damage by drinking less and adding, through food and supplementation, the nutrients alcohol destroys.

Since alcohol is a carbohydrate, to be metabolized it requires the B vitamins found in whole grains, brewer's yeast, or organic liver. Personally, I think it's a good idea to take a vitamin supplement for insurance. If you do, take the whole B-complex to maintain the proper balance, rather than separate B vitamins. If you drank heavily in the past and have greatly reduced your alcohol intake, don't use 100-milligram doses of B vitamins. Your liver, possibly damaged by excessive alcohol, has to work harder to utilize some of them. It is always safer to take lower potencies twice a day.

B_1 (thiamine) is one of the B vitamins that helps your body digest and assimilate the alcohol you drink. It also contributes to a healthy nervous system. Whenever you drink, your body uses more B_1, found naturally in brewer's yeast. If you're drinking regularly you need additional amounts through supplementation or yeast each day.

B_{12} and folic acid malabsorption commonly result from drinking and can lead to anemia. Found primarily in animal protein, B_{12} is difficult to absorb. If you have been told you are anemic, you may want to increase your intake of animal protein and take additional B_{12} in a B-complex formula. Pancreatic extracts have been used to help the body absorb B_{12} more readily. If you have anemia, you may not have enough B_{12} in your diet or you may have difficulty absorbing it. Glandular extracts of pancreas, found in health food stores, may enhance its absorption.

Alcohol interferes with your bones' ability to use folic acid, so even a diet of fresh vegetables, high in folates, could leave you depleted. I recommend you increase your vegetable and decrease your alcohol intake and take a supplement that includes B-complex.

Of all minerals, magnesium, needed most by women to assimilate calcium, is excreted more rapidly through the urine when you drink alcohol. Alcohol is a diuretic that increases the kidney's excretion, and magnesium deficiencies have been found in the muscles and blood of alcoholics. For drinking women, I use supplements with a reversed ratio of calcium to magnesium—two parts magnesium to one part calcium—like the multi-vitamin/mineral formula discussed in the beginning of this chapter. Whole grains, legumes, and dark green vegetables naturally contain magnesium, but if it is being eliminated from your body more quickly than usual, you will need to replenish it to prevent calcium-deficiency problems such as arthritis and premenstrual syndrome. If you have premenstrual mood swings and anxiety, magnesium would probably benefit you (see the Premenstrual Syndrome Diet).

Above all, pay attention to when and why you drink. If you're using alcohol to relax or feel more sociable, you are using it as a drug—be careful of drug abuse.

157

One or two drinks a day may seem innocent, but seven to fourteen drinks a week, thirty to sixty drinks a month, and four hundred to eight hundred drinks a year is not innocent at all.

Suggested Dietary Changes for the Social Drinker's Diet: The Anti-illness Diet is the foundation for this nutritional program, with an emphasis on whole grains, legumes, and green leafy vegetables. If you like liver, add organic liver every week or two for added B vitamins; or use brewer's yeast instead.

Supplements:

Multi-vitamin/mineral with more magnesium than calcium, to balance the increased magnesium excretion and supply you with adequate B vitamins.

50-milligram B-complex formula (rather than 100-milligram), two times a day

1 to 2 tablespoons brewer's yeast, sprinkled over cereal or salad

THE SMOKER'S DIET

Both active and passive smokers are affected by cigarette smoke. Passive smokers, people who live or work with smokers and cannot avoid inhaling their smoke, have more incidence of lung cancer than people who breathe smoke-free air. A study conducted in West Germany on passive smoking, reported in *Health and Longevity Report*, found 61.5 percent of the nonsmoking women who had lung cancer lived with smokers.

If you are either an active or passive smoker who is not ready, willing, or able to completely give up smoking, minimize the damage it causes by adding two important nutrients to your diet: vitamin C and beta carotene.

The Recommended Daily Allowance (RDA) for vitamin C in women is 45 milligrams. This means less than 45 milligrams can cause scurvy, a vitamin C–deficiency disease. One cigarette destroys 25 milligrams, and smoking a pack of cigarettes a day uses up 500 milligrams. An article on the need for increased vitamin C in smokers, published in *The Nutriton Report*, shows a two- to fourfold increase in vitamin C deficiency in smokers. Even if you have a cup of orange juice with breakfast and some tomatoes in your salad at lunch, it will not make up for the C lost through smoking. Taking vitamin C after each meal, when it is most easily absorbed, may be the best way for you to be sure you have enough of this important nutrient.

Beta carotene is not a new vitamin. It is a substance found in yellow plants, like corn, carrots, and sweet potatoes, that turns into vitamin A in the intestines. A diet rich in beta carotene has been found helpful in clearing the lungs of coal miners who inhale coal dust and of smokers with and without cancer.

I am not suggesting lung cancer can be cured by taking beta carotene, but the *International Clinical Nutrition Review* cites fifteen studies correlating lung cancer with a low intake of beta carotene and vice versa. Certainly this is enough reason to at least eat more foods rich in vitamin A. People who suffer from the effects of smog may also find relief by increasing carotene-rich foods or taking the vitamin in liquid or dried tablets, a more easily absorbed form than oil-based capsules.

Suggested Dietary Changes for the Smoker's Diet: Include as many foods high in vitamins C and A as you comfortably can. Fresh black currants and guavas contain large amounts of vitamin C, but if you don't have access to them, you can still get significant amounts from broccoli, brussel sprouts, cauliflower, collard greens, dandelion greens, grapefruit, kale, oranges, papayas, red and green bell peppers, parsley, and strawberries. Vitamin A is found in apricots, beet greens, broccoli, carrots, nectarines, pumpkins and yellow winter squash, spinach, and watermelon.

Supplements:

1000 milligrams vitamin C after each meal

20,000 iu beta carotene, two times a day

THE STRESSFUL LIVING DIET

More than 80 percent of the women I counsel name stress as one of the reasons for seeing me. They know that what they eat and drink isn't helping them, but do not know how much nutritional stress adds to their condition. If your lifestyle is stressful, you need to pay particularly close attention to what you eat and drink. The working woman is particularly vulnerable, as she is often surrounded by coffee, sugar, white flour, fatty foods, and alcohol. Fatigue, caused by the stress you're under and increased by the choice of foods around you, can result in your taking the path of least resistance and having a snack of coffee and sweet rolls, or grabbing a hamburger with french fries and a cola on the run. It's often easiest to eat whatever's available.

You may not be ready or able to eat well all of the time, particularly if you are a professional woman who travels, but even small changes are helpful in improving your health and reducing stress. If you are living a fast-paced life, unable to do much cooking for yourself and eating with people who go for rich or convenient foods, adopt the better-than approach: make the best choices you can to reduce your nutritional stress.

Cut back on those foods that have no nutritional value and that rob your body of vitamins, such as sugar, caffeine, alcohol, and white flour. Reduce fats, often used to excess in restaurant foods; ask for sauces on the side; use less butter; and pass on the cheese except in very small quantities.

Eat fresh vegetables, legumes, whole grains, and fish whenever you can. Salads of iceberg lettuce and a slice of hothouse tomato won't give you many nutrients, but dark green lettuce, spinach, cabbage, bean sprouts, broccoli, and zucchini, as well as legumes such as garbanzos and kidney beans, are common fare at many salad bars and replace vitamins and minerals depleted by stress. B vitamins, called antistress vitamins because they give support to the nervous system, are found in abundance in whole grains and fresh fish. Cornmeal, in the form of corn bread and corn tortillas, can be found in some restaurants, and coffee shops often serve oatmeal, a much-overlooked breakfast food. Go out of your way to eat these foods, especially if you drink, since alcohol destroys B vitamins. You may not find brown rice or millet on the menu, but look for restaurants that serve whole grain bread, rolls, or crackers.

Drink less alcohol by starting with Perrier or other mineral water. If you decide to have a drink later you may be able to limit yourself to one, rather than two or three. Choose something with ice that lasts a long time, like a white wine spritzer, and nurse it through your meal. If you like to unwind at night with a drink, switch to chamomile or another relaxing herb tea.

One real stress on your digestive system is overeating. Since most restaurants serve larger portions than you need at one sitting, eat only as much as you need to feel satisfied and take the rest home for the next day's lunch or dinner. Share an occasional dessert if you are not too full, but don't make it a regular part of dining out. Desserts usually contain too much sugar and fats.

Suggested Dietary Changes for The Stressful Living Diet:

Eliminate	Reduce	Emphasize
sugar	caffeine	fresh vegetables
	white flour	legumes
	fats	whole grains when possible
	alcohol	fish

Supplements:

Multi-vitamin/mineral

50-milligram B-complex after morning and noon meals

1000 milligrams vitamin C after each meal

80 milligrams raw adrenal tissue morning and noon after meals. Use these glandular supplements for a month or two during your more stressful times for additional support.

Auxiliary Treatment: Reduce stress through any method that will fit into your lifestyle. You may want to become more aware of some on-the-job stresses you may have overlooked. If so, *Healthy People in Unhealthy Places: Stress and Fitness at Work*, by Kenneth Pelletier, will provide you with interesting insights. Get more sleep, spend a few hours reading for relaxation, soak in a hot bath, listen to music, get away for an afternoon or a weekend whenever you can. The following can help reduce your total level of stress and result in more sustained energy.

Meditation and relaxation exercises: Five full minutes of quiet time twice a day will allow you to break your cycle of rushing around. Ten minutes of meditation, visualization, or relaxation techniques can take you to the calm center inside you, and twenty minutes to half an hour will leave you refreshed and able to resume work at a more relaxed, more effective pace. See the suggestions for books and tapes at the beginning of this chapter under the discussion of Auxiliary Treatments.

Massage: If you can afford it, have a massage on a regular basis. Whether it is once a week or once a month, you will soon find it is not a luxury, but a necessity. If you can't afford a professional massage, have a friend massage your back or feet. Once tense muscles begin to relax, you can focus on holding on to that feeling as long as possible.

Exercise: Regular moderate exercise from three to six times a week will energize and relax you. Yoga, stretching exercises, walking, biking, swimming, and jogging are some ways to limber your muscles and increase blood flow throughout your body. Be careful not to overexercise. A two-hour aerobics class might be a good way to shape up your body, but it can be an added stress if you're already overdoing it in other areas.

Psychotherapy: You may be under stress because you're stuck in a job or living situation that's not working for you. It can be more stressful to try to work out your problems by yourself than to speak with someone who is trained to help you see yourself clearly enough to find your own solutions. If you think you're too busy to go into therapy, this may be a form of resistance. Check it out. Reducing your emotional stress provides a great deal of extra energy.

AFTERWORD

GETTING HEALTHY,

STAYING HEALTHY

N ow you're on your way to good health. You have learned how to create a sound nutritional foundation using the Anti-illness Diet and you have been given suggestions to make it work. The questionnaires in chapter 3 revealed your inherited and accumulated strengths and weaknesses, and the specific diets in chapter 5 are designed to integrate easily into your basic program. I suggest you begin gradually, incorporating this dietary information at a comfortable pace. Be patient with yourself. Good health is a lifelong program—a program you can follow, and a program that changes as your body and needs change.

Begin now to create a team of health practitioners who can corroborate your condition and monitor your program. Health-care professionals are often excellent diagnosticians, good resources in emergencies, and often have a network of other reputable colleagues for referrals. It is much wiser to have someone else working with you than to be your own doctor.

Look for someone who understands and respects your desire to use good nutrition to overcome your health problems. Find a practitioner who understands you do not have to be clinically sick to have uncomfortable and unnecessary symptoms. Ask your friends for referrals, call or write to professional associations like those mentioned in this book, and ask the practitioners questions before making an appointment. Some of the questions you may want to ask include:

1. I want to become more knowledgable about my body and more responsible for my health than I've been before. Are you willing to be a partner with me in this?

2. I would like to understand your points of view and any findings from laboratory tests you may decide to run. Are you willing to spend a reasonable amount of time discussing them with me?

3. What is your opinion of using nutrition to overcome my health problems?

4. Are you willing to work with me if I choose to use natural methods as much as possible?

Like this book, the most a health practitioner can do is show you how to work with yourself. Many of the clues you need to do this are in your family's and your own health history, your symptoms, and your diet. Become familiar with your body and how it works so your activities and diet contribute to good health rather than detract from it. Ask questions and investigate each situation thoroughly until you understand why you are doing what you've been asked to do. I tell my patients there are no dumb questions, just areas that have never been explained to them,

Once you have become your own nutrition detective and understand why you're eating particular foods and avoiding others you can make any nutritional program work for you. Make those changes that make sense to you and look for explanations for those that don't. Take back the responsibility for your health you've given over to others, form a team with practitioners who are willing to be your allies, and give yourself the highest quality health you can.

REFERENCES AND RECOMMENDED READING

CHAPTER ONE

Abraham, Guy E. "The Calcium Controversy." *The Journal of Applied Nutrition*, Vol. 34, No. 2: pp. 69–73.

Abraham, Guy E. "Magnesium Deficiency in Premenstrual Tension." Magnesium-Bulletin, Vol. 4.

Airola, Paavo. *How to Get Well.* Phoenix, Ariz: Health Plus Publishers, 1974.

Alford, Betty B., and Bogle, Margaret L. *Nutrition During the Life Cycle.* Englewood Cliffs, N.J.: Prentice-Hall, Inc., 1982.

Barcus, Robert. "Milk: Not for Everyone." *Nutrition Action,* Vol. 8, No. 9: p. 14.

Bland, Jeffrey. "The Nutritional Supplement Analysis Laboratory of the Linus Pauling Institute of Science and Medicine." Palo Alto, Calif., 1984.

Brewster, Letitia, and Jacobson, Michael. "The Changing American Diet." Washington, D.C.: Center for Science in the Public Interest, 1983.

Pfeiffer, Carl C. *Mental and Elemental Nutrients: A Physician's Guide to Nutrition and Health Care.* New Canaan, Conn.: Keats Publishing Inc., 1975.

Shearman, Rodney P. *Human Reproductive Physiology,* 2nd ed. Oxford: Blackwell Scientific Publications, pp. 470–471.

Suitor, Carol West, and Hunter, Merrily Forbes. *Nutrition: Principles and Application in Health Promotion.* New York: J. B. Lippincott, 1980.

Tobin, Richard B., and Mehlman, Myron A., eds. *Advances in Human Nutrition.* Park Forest South, Ill.: Pathotox Publishers, Inc., p. 71.

Wahlqvist, Mark L., and Isaksson, Bjorn. "Training in Clinical Nutrition: Undergraduate and Postgraduate." *The Lancet,* Dec. 3, 1983: pp. 1295–1297.

Whitney, Eleanor Noss, and Cataldo, Corinne Balog. *Understanding Normal and Clinical Nutrition.* St. Paul, Minn.: West Publishing Co., 1983.

Williams, Roger J. *Nutrition Against Disease: Environmental Protection.* Huntington Beach, Calif.: International Institute of Natural Health Sciences, Inc.

Williams, Roger J., and Kalita, Dwight K., eds. *A Physician's Handbook on Orthomolecular Medicine.* New York: Pergamon Press, 1977.

CHAPTER TWO

Borrmann, Wm. R. *Comprehensive Guide to Nutrition,* 2nd ed., Chicago: New Horizons Publishing Company, 1979.

Forman, Robert. *How to Control Your Allergies.* New York: Larchmont Books, 1979.

Kirschmann, John D. *Nutrition Almanac.* New York: McGraw-Hill, 1979.

Mandell, Marshall, and Scanlon, Lynne Waller. *Dr Mandell's 5-Day Allergy Relief System.* New York: Pocket Books, 1979.

CHAPTER THREE

Alsleben, H. Rudolph, and Shute, Wilfrid E. *How to Survive the New Health Catastrophes.* Anaheim, Calif.: Survival Publications, Inc., 1973.

Bailey, Covert. *Fit or Fat?* Boston: Houghton Mifflin Co., 1978.

Bolton, Sanford; Null, Gary; and Pressman, Alan H. "Caffeine: Its Effects, Uses and Abuses." *The Journal of Applied Nutrition,* Vol. 33, No. 1.

Borrmann, Wm. R. *Comprehensive Guide to Nutrition,* 2nd ed. Chicago: New Horizons Publishing Corporation, 1979.

"Caffeine and Health." *Nutrition and the M.D.,* Vol. 9, No. 8.

Correa, Pelayo. "Passive Smokers at Risk from Lung Cancer." *International Clinical Nutrition Review,* Vol. 4, No. 2.

Crook, William G. *The Yeast Connection.* Jacksonville, Tenn.: Professional Books, 1983.

"Effect of Alcohol on the Foetus." *International Clinical Nutrition Review,* Vol. 3, No. 4.

Goodman, Alfred; Goodman, Louis S.; and Gilman, Alfred. *The Pharmacological Basis of Therapeutics,* 6th edition. New York: Macmillan Publishing Co., 1980.

Guyton, Arthur C. *Textbook of Medical Physiology,* 4th ed. Philadelphia: W. B. Saunders Company, 1971.

Hargrove, J., and Abraham, Guy E. "The Incidence of Premenstrual Tension in a Gynecologic Clinic." *Journal of Reproductive Medicine,* 1982.

Lamott, Kenneth. *Escape from Stress.* New York: G. P. Putnam's Sons, 1975.

Lauersen, Niels, and Stukane, Eileen. *Listen to Your Body.* New York: Berkley Books, 1982.

Passwater, Richard A. "A Multi-Disciplinary View of Herpes Simplex II." *The Journal of Energy Medicine,* Vol. 1.

Roe, Daphne A. *Drug-Induced Nutritional Deficiencies.* Westport, Conn.: Avi Publishing Company, Inc., 1980.

Selye, Hans. *Stress Without Distress.* New York: New American Library, 1974.

Trevathan, Edwin; Layde, Peter; Webster, Linda A.; et al. "Smoking and Cancer of the Cervix." *International Clinical Nutrition Review,* Vol. 4, No. 2.

Truss, C. Orian. *The Missing Diagnosis.* Birmingham, Ala.: privately published, 1982.

Walther, David S. "Applied Kinesiology." Pueblo, Colo.: Systems DC, 1976.

CHAPTER FOUR

"Ad for 'Healthful' New Sweetener Mum on Saccharin Content." *Nutrition Action.* Washington, D.C.: The Center for Science in the Public Interest, April, 1984.

Alsleben, H. Rudolph, and Shute, Wilfrid E. *How to Survive the New Health Catastrophes.* Anaheim, Calif.: Survival Publications, Inc., 1973.

"Aluminum Exposure and Neurological Abnormalities." *International Clinical Nutrition Review,* Vol. 3, No. 4.

"Aluminum Toxicity." *International Clinical Nutrition Review,* Vol. 3, No. 4.

Bland, Jeffrey. *Your Health Under Siege: Using Nutrition to Fight Back.* Battleboro, Vt.: Stephen Greene Press, 1981.

Bolton, Sanford; Null, Gary; and Pressman, Alan H. "Caffeine: Its Effects, Uses and Abuses." *The Journal of Applied Nutrition,* Vol. 33, No. 1.

"Caffeine and Health." *Nutrition and the M.D.,* Vol. 9, No. 8: pp. 6–7.

Cheraskin, E., and Ringsdorf, W. M., Jr., with Brecher, Arline. *Psychodietetics: Food as the Key to Emotional Health.* New York: Stein and Day, 1974.

Culbreth, David M. R. *A Manual of Materia Medica and Pharmacology.* Philadelphia: Lea & Febiger, 1927.

Dadd, Debra Lynn. *Nontoxic & Natural.* Los Angeles: Jeremy P. Tarcher, 1984.

"Does Sugar Consumption Influence Breast Cancer?" *The Nutrition Report,* Vol. 1, No. 2.

Dusky, Lorraine, and Watson, Rita E. "Conquerable Cancer." *Town and Country,* May 1980: pp. 95–97.

Fieldman, Anita. "Frances Moore Lappe: The Next Step." *Whole Life Times,* July– Aug., 1984.

Ford, Marjorie Winn; Hillyard, Susan; and Koock, Mary Faulk. *The Deaf Smith Country Cookbook.* New York: Collier Books, 1973.

Fritch, Albert J., ed. *The Household Pollutants Guide.* New York: Anchor Books, Center for Science in the Public Interest, 1978.

Gordon, T., and Kannel, W. B. "Drinking and its relation to smoking, BP, blood lipids, and uric acid. The Framingham Study." Nutrition abstracts and reviews, Series A, Vol. 54, No. 2–3.

Hausman, Patricia. *Jack Sprat's Legacy: The Science and Politics of Fat and Cholesterol.* New York: Richard Marek Publishers, 1981.

Horrobin, David F., and Phil, D. "The Importance of Gamma-Linolenic Acid and Prostaglandin El in Human Nutrition and Medicine." *Journal of Holistic Medicine,* Vol. 3, No. 2.

Hunter, Beatrice Trum. *Fact/Book on Food Additives and Your Health.* New Canaan, Conn.: Keats Publishing, 1972.

"Increased Permeability of Blood-Brain Barrier Due to Aluminum." *International Clinical Nutrition Review,* Vol. 4, No. 3.

"Is Peanut Oil Atherogenic?" *International Clinical Nutrition Review,* Vol. 4, No. 3.

Kirschmann, John D. *Nutrition Almanac.* New York: McGraw-Hill, 1979.

Liebman, Bonnie F., and Moyer, Greg. "Sugar: How Safe is It?" *Nutrition Action,* Washington, D.C.: Center for Science in the Public Interest, reprint, 1981.

Morck, T.A.; Lynch, S. R.; and Cook, J. D. "Inhibition of Food Iron Absorption by Coffee." *International Clinical Nutrition Review,* Vol. 3, No. 4.

Newell, Guy R., and Ellison, Neil M., eds. "Nutrition and Cancer: Etiology and Treatment." *Progress in Cancer Research and Therapy,* Vol. 17; New York: Raven Press, 1981.

Reuben, David. *The Save-Your-Life Diet: High-Fiber Protection from Six of the Most Serious Diseases of Civilization.* New York: Random House, 1975.

CHAPTER FIVE

Bland, Jeffrey, and Presbo, Eric. "Vitamin E: Comparative Absorption Studies." *International Clinical Nutrition Review,* Vol. 4, No. 2.

Davis, Adelle. *Let's Get Well.* New York: Harcourt, Brace & World, 1965.

Kirschmann, John D. *Nutrition Almanac,* revised ed. New York: McGraw-Hill, 1979.

MacHovec, Frank J. *Om, A Guide to Meditation and Inner Tranquility.* White Plains, N.Y.: Peter Pauper Press, 1973.

Marshall, John. L., with Barbash, Heather. *The Sports Doctor's Fitness Book for Women.* New York: Dell Trade Paperback, 1981.

Nittler, Alan H. "DNA-RNA Glandular and Tissue Specificity." *The Journal of the Nutritional Academy of Nutritional Consultants,* Vol. 1, No. 1.

Schmitt, Walter H., Jr. "Common Glandular Dysfunctions in the General Practice." Chapel Hill, N.C.: privately published, 1981.

Simonton, O. Carl, M.D.; Matthews-Simonton, Stephanie; and Creighton, James L. *Getting Well Again.* New York: Bantam Books, 1978.

"Vitamin C Bioavailability." *International Clinical Nutrition Review,* Vol. 4, No. 4.

THE RECOVERING ALCOHOLIC'S DIET

Alsleben, H. Rudolph, and Shute, Wilfrid E. *How to Survive the New Health Catastrophes.* Anaheim, Calif.: Survival Publications, 1973.

Baker, H., and Frank, O. "A Vitamin Profile of Metabolic Disturbances." *The Journal of Applied Nutrition, Vol. 33, No. 1.*

Dworkin, Brad M., and Rosenthal, William S. "Selenium and the Alcoholic." *The Lancet,* Vol. 1, No. 8384.

Halsted, Charles H. "Nutritional Implications of Alcohol." *Nutrition Reviews' Present Knowledge in Nutrition,* 4th ed. Washington, D.C.: The Nutrition Foundation, 1976.

Ketcham, Katherine, and Mueller, L. Ann *Eating Right to Live Sober.* Seattle: Madrona Publishers, 1983.

Kirschmann, John D. *Nutrition Almanac,* revised ed. New York: McGraw-Hill, 1979.

Korsten, Mark A., and Lieber, Charles S. "Nutrition and the Alcoholic." *Medical Clinics of North America,* Vol. 63, No. 5.

Poulos, C. Jean; Stoddard, Donald; and Carron, Kathryn. *The Relationship of Stress to Hypoglycemia and Alcoholism.* Huntington Beach, Calif.: International Institute of Natural Health Sciences, 1976.

Roe, Daphne A. *Drug-Induced Nutritional Deficiencies.* Westport, Conn.: AVI Publishing Co., 1980.

"Selenium and Acute Alcoholism." *International Clinical Nutrition Review,* Vol. 4, No. 3.

"Selenium Content of Specific Foods." *International Clinical Nutrition Review,* Vol. 4, No. 3.

"The Role of Nutritional Therapy in Alcoholism Treatment." *International Clinical Nutrition Review,* Vol. 4, No. 1.

Williams, Roger J. *Nutrition Against Disease.* Huntington Beach, Calif.: International Institute of Natural Health Sciences.

Williams, Roger J. *The Prevention of Alcoholism Through Nutrition.* New York: Bantam Books, 1981.

Williams, Roger J., and Kalita, Dwight K. eds. *A Physician's Handbook on Ortho-molecular Medicine.* New York: Pergamon Press, 1977.

THE FOOD ALLERGY DIET

Aas, Kjell. "Antigens in Food." *Nutrition Reviews,* Vol. 42, No. 3.

"Adverse Reactions to Food." *The Lancet,* Vol. 1, No. 8382.

Coca, Arthur F. *The Pulse Test.* New York: Lyle Stuart, 1959.

"Eliminate Your Allergies." *Health and Longevity Report,* Vol. 1, No. 10.

Forman, Robert. *How to Control Your Allergies.* New York: Larchmont Books, 1979.

Hills, Hilda Cherry. *Good Food, Gluten Free.* New Canaan, Conn.: Keats Publishing, 1976.

Jones, Marjorie Hurt. *The Allergy Self-Help Cookbook.* Emmaus, Pa.: Rodale Press, 1984.

Levin, Alan S., and Zellerbach, Merla. *The Type 1/Type 2 Allergy Relief Program,* Los Angeles: Jeremy P. Tarcher, 1983.

Mandell, Fran Gare. *Dr. Mandell's Allergy-Free Cookbook.* New York: Pocket Books, 1981.

Mandell, Marshall, and Scanlon, Lynne Waller. *Dr. Mandell's 5-Day Allergy Relief System.* New York: Pocket Books, 1979.

May, Charles D. "Food Sensitivity: Facts and Fancies." *Nutrition Reviews,* Vol. 42, No. 3.

Nonken, Pamela P., and Hirsch, S. Roger. *The Allergy Cookbook and Food-Buying Guide.* New York: Warner Books, 1982.

Philpott, William H., and Kalita, Dwight K. *Brain Allergies: The Psycho-Nutrient Connection.* New Canaan, Conn.: Keats Publishing, 1980.

Walther, David S. "Applied Kinesiology." Pueblo, Colo.: Systems DC, 1976.

Williams, Roger J., and Kalita, Dwight K., eds. *A Physician's Handbook on Ortho-molecular Medicine.* New York: Pergamon Press, 1977.

THE ARTHRITIS DIET

Antill, Ellen. "Arthritis: There's a War Going on and Your Health Is at Stake." *Health and Longevity Report,* Vol. 2, No. 10.

Blake, D. R., and Scott, D.G.I. "Assessment of Iron Deficiency in Rheumatoid Arthritis." *British Medical Journal,* Feb. 29, 1980.

Childers, Norman F., and Russo, Gerard M. *The Nightshades and Health.* Somerville, N.J.: Somerset Press, 1977.

Fredericks, Carlton. *Arthritis: Don't Learn to Live with It.* New York: Grosset & Dunlap, 1981.

Fredericks, Carlton. *Dr. Carlton Frederick's New and Complete Nutrition Handbook.* Huntington Beach, Calif.: International Institute of Natural Health Sciences, 1976.

Kowsari, Badri; Finnie, Sheryl K.; Carter, Randolph L.; Love, James; Katz, Paul; Longley, Sheldon; and Panush, Richard S. "Assessment of the Diet of Patients with Rheumatoid Arthritis and Osteoarthritis." *Journal of the American Dietetic Assn.,* Vol. 82, No. 6.

Krause, Marie V. *Food, Nutrition and Diet Therapy,* 5th ed., Philadelphia: W. B. Saunders Co., 1979.

Panush, R. S.; Carter, R. L.; Katz, P.; Kowsari, B.; Longley, S.; and Finnie, S. "Diet Therapy for Rheumatoid Arthritis." *Arthritis Rheum,* Vol. 26, No. 4.

Parke, A. L., and Hughes, G.R.V. "Rheumatoid Arthritis and Food: A Case Study." *British Medical Journal,* June 20, 1981.

Pfeiffer, Carl C. *Mental and Elemental Nutrients.* New Canaan, Conn.: Keats Publishing, 1975.

Schmitt, Walter H., Jr. "Common Glandular Dysfunctions in the General Practice." Chapel Hill, N. C.: 1981.

Scott, D. L., Farr, M.; Hawkins, C. F.; Wilkinson, R.; and Bold, A. M. "Serum Calcium Levels in Rheumatoid Arthritis." *Annual Rheum Disease,* Vol. 40, No. 6.

Williams, Roger J. *Nutrition Against Disease.* New York: Bantam Books, 1971.

Williams, Roger J., and Kalita, Dwight K., eds. *A Physician's Handbook on Ortho-molecular Medicine.* New York: Pergamon Press, 1977.

Wright, Jonathan V. *Dr. Wright's Book of Nutritional Therapy.* Emmaus, Pa.: Rodale Press, 1979.

Ziff, Morris. "Diet in the Treatment of Rheumatoid Arthritis." *Arthritis and Rheumatism,* Vol. 26, No. 4.

THE BLOOD SUGAR DIET

Biermann, June, and Toohey, Barbara. *The Diabetic's Total Health Book.* Los Angeles: Jeremy P. Tarcher, 1980.

Biermann, June, and Toohey, Barbara. *The Peripatetic Diabetic.* Los Angeles: Jeremy P. Tarcher, 1984.

Bland, Jeffrey. *Your Health Under Siege: Using Nutrition to Fight Back.* Brattle-boro, Vt.: Stephen Greene Press, 1981.

Bland, Jeffrey, ed. *Medical Applications of Clinical Nutrition.* New Canaan, Conn.: Keats Publishing, 1983.

Buist, R. A. "Metabolic Responses to Different Physical 'Forms' of Food." *The Lancet,* Vol. 3, No. 4.

"Effect of Processing on Digestibility and the Blood Glucose Response: A Study on Lentils." *The Lancet,* Vol. 3, No. 4.

Fuchs, Nan. "A Holistic Approach to the Diagnosis and Treatment of Hypo-glycemia," doctoral dissertation, 1982.

Goodhart, Robert S., and Shils, Maurice E., eds. *Modern Nutrition in Health and Disease,* 6th ed. Philadelphia: Lea & Febiger, 1980.

Jenkins, David J. A. "Dietary Carbohydrates and Their Glycemic Responses." *Journal of the American Medical Assn.,* Vol. 251, No. 21.

Jenkins, David J. A.; Wolever, Thomas M. S.; Jenkins, Alexandra L.; Josse, Robert G.; and Wong, Gerald S. "The Glycemic Response to Carbohydrate Foods." *The Lancet,* Vol. 2, No. 8399.

Krause, Marie V. *Food, Nutrition and Diet Therapy,* 5th ed. Philadelphia: W. B. Saunders Co., 1979.

Madill, Peter. "Hypoglycemia, Stress and Psychosomatic Illness: The Roll of Elec-troacupuncture According to Voll." *American Journal of Acupuncture,* Vol. 8, No. 2.

Mertz, Walter. "Chromium and Its Relation to Carbohydrate Metabolism." *Medical Clinics of North America,* Vol. 60, No. 4.

Nutrition Reviews' Present Knowledge in Nutrition, 4th ed. New York: Nutrition Foundation, 1976.

Pfeiffer, Carl C. *Mental and Elemental Nutrients.* New Canaan, Conn.: Keats Publishing, 1975.

Poulos, C. Jean; Stoddard, Donald; and Cannon, Kathryn. *The Relationship of Stress to Hypoglycemia and Alcoholism.* Huntington Beach, Calif.: International Institute of Natural Health Sciences, 1976.

Vitale, Joseph J., and Broitman, Selwyn A., eds. *Advances in Human Clinical Nutrition.* Massachusetts: John Wright, PSG, 1982.

"Vitamin C and Diabetes Millitus." *The Lancet,* Vol. 4, No. 3.

Williams, Roger J., and Kalita, Dwight K., eds. *A Physician's Handbook on Ortho-molecular Medicine.* New York: Pergamon Press, 1977.

Wright, Jonathan V. *Dr. Wright's Book of Nutritional Therapy.* Emmaus, Pa.: Rodale Press, 1979.

THE GOOD DIGESTION DIET

Alsleben, H. Rudolph, and Shute, Wilfrid E. *How to Survive the New Health Catastrophes.* Anaheim, Calif.: Survival Publications, 1973.

"Balancing Body Chemistry with Nutrition Seminars." Geneva, Ohio: AK Printing, 1984.

Borrmann, Wm. R. *Comprehensive Guide to Nutrition,* 2nd ed. Chicago: New Horizons Publishing Corp., 1979.

Kirschmann, John D. *Nutrition Almanac,* revised ed. New York: McGraw-Hill, 1979.

Schmitt, Walter H., Jr. "Common Glandular Dysfunctions in the General Practice." Chapel Hill, N.C.: privately published, 1981.

Schmitt, Walter H., Jr., "Compiled Notes on Clinical Nutritional Products." Private-ly published, 1979.

Walther, David S. "Applied Kinesiology." Pueblo, Colo.: Systems DC, 1976.

THE HEADACHE DIET

Borrmann, Wm. R. *Comprehensive Guide to Nutrition,* 2nd ed. Chicago: New Horizons Publishing Corp., 1979.

"Certain Foods Provoke Migraine." *Nutrition Reviews,* Vol. 42, No. 2.

Hanington, Edda. "Diet and Migraine." *Journal of Human Nutrition,* Vol. 34, No. 3.

Kirschmann, John D. *Nutrition Almanac,* revised ed. New York: McGraw-Hill, 1979.

McGough, Genevieve. "Food, Mood, Fate Generate Headaches." *Health and Longevity Report,* Vol. 2, No. 2.

Monro, Jean; Carini, Claudio; Brostoff, Jonathan; and Zilkha, K. "Food Allergy in Migraine." *The Lancet,* Vol. 2, No. 8184.

Pfeiffer, Carl C. *Mental and Elemental Nutrients.* New Canaan, Conn.: Keats Publishing, 1975.

Saper, Joel R., and Magee, Kenneth R. *Freedom from Headaches.* New York: Simon and Schuster, 1978.

Stern, Judith S. "Meals and Migraine." *Vogue,* March 1984.

Wright, Jonathan V. *Dr. Wright's Book of Nutritional Therapy.* Emmaus, Pa.: Rodale Press, 1979.

THE STRONG IMMUNE SYSTEM DIET

Beisel, William R.; Edelman, Robert; Nauss, Kathleen; and Suskind, Robert M. "Single-Nutrient Effects on Immunologic Functions." *The Journal of the American Medical Assn.,* Vol. 245, No. 1.

Bland, Jeffrey. *Your Health Under Siege: Using Nutrition to Fight Back.* Brattle-boro, Vt.: Stephen Greene Press, 1981.

"Cigarette Smoking Causes Immunosuppression." *International Clinical Nutrition Review,* Vol. 4, No. 2.

Chandra, R.K.; Joshi, P.; Au, B.; Woodford, G.; and Chandra, S. "Nutrition and Immunocompetence of the Elderly." *Nutrition Research,* Vol. 2, No. 3.

Chandra, Ranjit Kumar. "Nutrition, Immunity, and Infection: Present Knowledge and Future Directions." *The Lancet,* Vol 1, No. 8326.

Goodhart, Robert S., and Shils, Maurice E. *Modern Nutrition in Health and Disease,* 6th ed. Philadelphia: Lea & Febiger, 1980.

Kaslow, Arthur L., and Miles, Richard B. *Freedom from Chronic Disease.* Los Angeles: Jeremy P. Tarcher, 1979.

Levin, Alan Scott, and Zellerbach, Merla. *The Type 1/Type 2 Allergy Relief Program.* Los Angeles: Jeremy P. Tarcher, 1983.

"Low-Fat Diet Enhances Immune System." *The Nutrition Report,* Vol. 2, No. 5.

"Thymosin Opening New Vistas in the Search for Quality Aging." *Health and Longevity Report,* Vol. 2, No. 7.

Walford, Roy L. *Maximum Life Span.* New York: Avon Books, 1983.

Williams, Roger J., and Kalita, Dwight K. eds. *A Physician's Handbook on Ortho-molecular Medicine.* New York: Pergamon Press, 1977.

THE HEALTHY SKIN DIET:

Bland, Jeffrey. *Medical Applications of Clinical Nutrition.* New Canaan, Conn.: Keats Publishing, 1983.

Bland, Jeffrey, and Prestbo, Eric. "Vitamin E: Comparison Absorption Studies." *International Clinical Nutrition Review,* Vol. 4, No. 2.

Fuchs, N.; Hakim, M.; and Abraham, Guy E. "The Effect of a Nutritional Supplement, Optivite for Women, on Liver Function Tests and Midluteal Serum Steroid Levels in Women with Premenstrual Tension Syndromes." Submitted to the *Journal of the American College of Nutrition.*

Kirschmann, John D. *Nutrition Almanac,* revised ed. New York: McGraw-Hill, 1979.

Kunin, Richard A. *Mega-Nutrition for Women.* New York: McGraw-Hill, 1983.

Wright, Jonathan V. *Dr. Wright's Book of Nutritional Therapy.* Emmaus, Pa.: Rodale Press, 1979.

THE ANOREXIA DIET

"Anorexia Nervosa: The Starving Disease." Grover City, Calif.: Anorexia Nervosa and Related Eating Disorders (AN/RED), newsletter.

Beaumont, P.J.; Chambers, T. L.; Rouse, L.; and Abraham, S. F.; "The Diet Composition and Nutritional Knowledge of Patients with Anorexia Nervosa." *Journal of Human Nutrition,* Vol. 35, No. 4.

Bryce-Smith, D., and Simpson, R.I.D. "Case of Anorexia Nervosa Responding to Zinc Sulphate." *The Lancet,* Vol. 2, No. 8398.

Golden, Neville, and Sacker, Ira M. "An Overview of the Etiology, Diagnosis, and Management of Anorexia Nervosa." *Clinical Pediatrics,* Vol. 111, No. 37.

Haller, Edwin W., and Cotton, Gerald E., eds. *Nutrition in the Young and the Elderly.* Lexington, Mass.: Collamore Press, 1983.

Horrobin, D. F., and Connane, S. C. "Interactions Between Zinc, Essential Fatty Acids and Prostaglandins: Relevance to Acrodermatitis Enteropathica, Total Parenteral Nutrition, the Glucagonoma Syndrome, Diabetes, Anorexia Nervosa, and Sickle Cell Anemia." *Medical Hypotheses,* Vol. 6, No. 3.

Schwabe, Arthur D., Lippe, Barbara M.; Chang, R. Jeffrey; Pops, Martin A.; and Yager, Joel. "Anorexia Nervosa: UCLA Conference." *Annals of Internal Medicine,* March 1981.

"Treatment Goal for Anorexia: Nutritional Rehabilitation." *American Family Physician,* June 1980.

THE BULEMIA AND COMPULSIVE-EATING DIET

"Anorexia Nervosa and Related Eating Disorders." Grover City, Calif.: AN/RED Alert Newsletter, March 1982.

Brenner, Marie. "Bulimarexia." *Savvy Magazine,* June 1980.

"Bulemia: A Rage to Fill." American Anorexia Nervosa Association Newsletter, Vol. 5, No. 2. (133 Cedar Lane, Teaneck, N.J. 07666; (201) 836–1800).

Harris, Robert T. "Bulimarexia and Related Serious Eating Disorders with Medical Complications." *Annals of Internal Medicine,* Vol. 3, No. 11.

McLaughlin, Loretta. "New Theories on Weighty Matters Concerning Obesity." *Los Angeles Times,* March 4, 1984.

Orbach, Susie. *Fat Is a Feminist Issue.* New York: Berkley Publishing, 1978.

Rudnick, F. David, "Medical and Neurological Aspects of Bulimia." *Binge Eating and Purging: Recognition of Bulimia.* UCLA symposium, Los Angeles, Calif., June 26, 1982.

Yager, Joel, M.D. "The Spectrum of Bulimic Disorders: An Overview and Typical Cases." *Binge Eating and Purging: Recognition and Management of Bulimia,* UCLA symposium, Los Angeles, Calif., June 16, 1982.

THE AMENORRHEA DIET

"Amenorrhea Associated with Carotenaemia." *Journal of the American Medical Assn.,* Vol. 249, No. 7: pp. 926–928.

Baxter, Kevin. "Women's Running." *Runner's World,* August, 1983.

Frisch, Rose E. "Amenorrhea, Vegetarianism, and/or Low Fat?" *The Lancet,* Vol. 1, No. 8384.

Grieve, M. *A Modern Herbal.* New York: Dover Publications, 1971.

Hsu, Hong-yen, and Easer, Douglas H. *For Women Only: Chinese Herbal Formulas.* Taiwan: Oriental Healing Arts Institute, 1982.

"Menstrual Cycle Dysfunction and Prolonged Strenuous Exercise in Women." *International Clinical Nutrition Review,* Vol. 3, No. 4.

Miller, Sue. "Women Athletes and Menstruation." *Los Angeles Times,* December 7, 1983.

Thomson, J. A., and Ratcliffe, W. A. "Dietary Amenorrhoea and Subclinical Hypothyroidism with Elevated TSH Responsive to Weight Gain." *Postgraduate Medical Journal,* Vol. 56, No. 660.

THE CANDIDA ALBICANS DIET

Crook, William G. *The Yeast Connection,* 2nd ed. Jackson, Tenn.: Professional Books, 1983.

"Dietary Suppression of Candida Albicans." Pompano Beach, Fla. 33060: Life Care Center, privately published.

Susser, Murray; Rowland, Karen; and Newcomer, Mari. "Preliminary Study on Homeopathic Candida Dilution Therapy." Oklahoma City: Bio-Genesis Medical Center, privately published.

Truss, C. Orion. *The Missing Diagnosis.* Birmingham, Ala.: 1983.

Truss, C. Orion. "Restoration of Immunologic Competence to Candida Albicans." *The Journal of Orthomolecular Psychiatry,* Vol. 9, No. 4: pp. 17–37.

Truss, C. Orion. "The Role of Candida Albicans in Human Illness." *The Journal of Orthomolecular Psychiatry,* Vol. 10, No. 4: pp. 228–238.

THE CYST AND TUMOR DIET

"Breast Cancer Linked With Sugar." *East West Journal,* July 1983.

Brooks, Philip G.; Gart, Sandi; Helfond, Alfred J.; Margolin, Malcolm L.; and Allen, Arthur S. "Measuring the Effect of Caffeine Restriction on Fibrocystic Breast Disease." *The Journal of Reproductive Medicine,* Vol. 26, No. 6.

"Does Sugar Consumption Influence Breast Cancer?" *The Nutrition Report,* Vol. 1, No. 2.

Garrison, Robert, Jr. "Dietary Fat and Breast Cancer: Can We Afford to Wait?" *The Nutrition Report,* Vol. 2, No. 5.

Gonzalez, Elizabeth Rasche. "Vitamin E Relieves Most Cystic Breast Disease; May Alter Lipids, Hormones." *Journal of the American Medical Assn.,* Vol. 244, No. 10.

Goodhart, Robert S., and Shils, Maurice E. *Modern Nutrition in Health and Disease,* 6th ed. Philadelphia: Lea & Febiger, 1978.

Napoli, Maryann. "Breast Cancer: An Update." *Network News.* Washington, D.C., Vol. 8, No. 4.

THE HERPES DIET

Kaslof, Leslie J., ed. *Wholistic Dimensions in Healing, A Resource Guide.* New York: Doubleday, 1978.

Lauersen, Niels, and Stukane, Eileen. *Listen to Your Body.* New York: Berkley Books, 1982.

Ozonoff, David. "A Multi-Disciplinary View of Herpes Simplex II." *The Journal of Energy Medicine,* Vol. 1.

Passwater, Richard. "L-Lysine Stops Herpes and Other Viruses." *Nutrition Consultant,* Sept./Oct. 1980.

THE MENOPAUSE DIET

Biskind, Morton S.; Biskind, Gerson R.; and Biskind, Leonard H. "Nutritional Deficiency in the Etiology of Menorrhagia, Metrorrhagia, Cystic Mastitis, and Premenstrual Tension." *Surg. Gynecol. Obstet.,* Vol. 78, No. 49.

Boston Women's Health Book Collective. *Our Bodies, Ourselves.* New York: Simon and Schuster, 1979.

Diagram Group. *Woman's Body: An Owner's Manual.* New York: Paddington Press Ltd., 1977.

Greenwood, Sadja. *Menopause, Naturally.* San Francisco: Volcano Press, 1984.

Laiken, Deidre S. *Beautiful Body Building.* New York: The New American Library, 1979.

Marshall, John L., with Barbash, Heather. *The Sports Doctor's Fitness Book for Women.* New York: Dell Trade Paperback, 1981.

Reitz, Rosetta. *Menopause, A Positive Approach.* England: Penguin Books, 1977.

Schmitt, Walter H., Jr. "Common Glandular Dysfunctions in the General Practice." Chapel Hill, N.C.: privately published, 1981.

Zimmer, Susan. "Nutrition and Older Women." *Network News.* Washington, D.C., March/April 1984.

THE MENSTRUAL CRAMPS DIET

Abraham, Guy E. "Nutrition and the Premenstrual Tension Syndrome." *Journal of Applied Nutrition,* Sept. 1984.

Horrobin, David F. "The Importance of Gamma-Linolenic Acid and Prostaglandin El in Human Nutrition and Medicine." *Journal of Holistic Medicine,* Vol. 3, No. 2.

Hutchens, Alma R. *Indian Herbology of North America.* London: Garden City Press Ltd., 1973.

Perlmutter, Cathy. "The No-More Pain Guide to Your Menstrual Cycle." *Spring,* Jan./Feb. 1983.

Ritz, Sandra. "How to Deal with Menstrual Cramps." *Medical Self-Care,* spring 1981.

Schmitt, Walter H., Jr., "Common Glandular Dysfunctions in the General Practice." Chapel Hill, N. C.: privately published, 1981.

THE OSTEOPOROSIS DIET

Abraham, Guy E. "The Calcium Controversy." *Journal of Applied Nutrition,* Vol. 34, No. 2.

Abraham, Guy E. "Nutrition and the Premenstrual Tension Syndromes." *Journal of Applied Nutrition,* Sept. 1984.

Bland, Jeffrey S. "Diet and Bone Status." *The Nutrition Report,* March 1984.

Briscoe, Anne M., and Ragan, Charles. "Effect of Magnesium on Calcium Metabolism in Man." *The American Journal of Clinical Nutrition,* Vol. 19, No. 5.

"Calcium and Exercise Prevent Osteoporosis." *Today's Living,* August 1983.

Colimore, Benjamin, and Colimore, Sarah Stewart. *Nutrition and Your Body.* Los Angeles: Light Wave Press, 1974.

Goodhart, Robert S., and Shils, Maurice E. *Modern Nutrition in Health and Disease,* 6th ed. Philadelphia: Lea & Febiger, 1978.

Johnson, Sharon. "Women Cautioned on Health Matters." *Los Angeles Times,* April 12, 1984.

Juan, David. "The Clinical Importance of Hypomagnesemia." *Surgery,* Vol. 91, No. 5.

Laakso, Ulla Kristiina. "Are You Getting Enough Calcium?" *Nutrition Health Review,* spring 1984.

Linkswiler, Hellen M. *Nutrition Reviews' Present Knowledge in Nutrition,* 4th ed. New York: The Nutrition Foundation, 1976.

MacPherson, Kathleen. "Is Osteoporosis Inevitable?" *Network News.* Washington, D.C., March/April 1984.

Massey, Linda K., and Wise, Kevin J. "The Effect of Dietary Caffeine on Urinary Excretion of Calcium, Magnesium, Sodium and Potassium in Healthy Young Females." *Nutrition Research,* Vol. 4.

Oyster, Nancy; Morton, Max; and Linnell, Sheri. "Physical Activity and Osteoporosis in Post-Menopausal Women." *Medicine and Science in Sports and Exercise,* Vol. 16, No. 1.

Taylor, Keith B., and Luean, E. *Clinical Nutrition.* New York: McGraw-Hill, 1983.

THE PREGNANCY DIET

"Association of Maternal Smoking with Body Composition of the Newborn." *International Clinical Review,* Vol. 4, No. 3.

Bland, Jeffrey S. "Seminar Notes." Overland Park, Kansas: International Academy of Preventative Medicine, privately published.

Bland, Jeffrey. *Your Health Under Siege: Using Nutrition to Fight Back.* Battleboro, Vt.: Stephen Greene Press, 1981.

"Effect of Alcohol on the Foetus." *International Clinical Nutrition Review,* Vol. 3, No. 4.

Goodhart, Robert S., and Shils, Maurice E. *Modern Nutrition in Health and Disease,* 6th ed. Philadelphia: Lea & Febiger, 1980.

Kirschmann, John D. *Nutrition Almanac,* revised ed. New York: McGraw-Hill, 1979.

Mahan, Charles S. "Revolution in Obstetrics: Pregnancy Nutrition." *Journal of the Florida Medical Assn.,* April 1979.

Nutrition Reviews' Present Knowledge in Nutrition, 4th ed. New York: The Nutrition Foundation, 1976.

Roe, Daphne A. *Drug-Induced Nutritional Deficiencies.* Westport, Conn.: AVI Publishing Co. 1976.

Williams, Roger J. *Nutrition Against Disease.* Huntington Beach, Calif.: International Institute of Natural Health Sciences.

Williams, Roger J., and Kalita, Dwight K. eds. *A Physician's Handbook on Orthomolecular Medicine.* New York: Pergamon Press, 1977.

Wright, Jonathan V. *Dr. Wright's Book of Nutritional Therapy.* Emmaus, Pa.: Rodale Press, 1979.

THE PREMENSTRUAL SYNDROME DIET

Abraham, Guy E. "Nutrition and the Premenstrual Syndrome." *Journal of Applied Nutrition,* Sept. 1984.

Abraham, Guy E. "Protol for a PMT Clinic." Privately published.

Alsleben, H. Rudolph, and Shute, Wilfrid E. *How to Survive the New Health Catastrophes.* Anaheim, Calif.: Survival Publications, 1973.

Fuchs, N.; Hakim, M.; and Abraham, G. E. "The Effect of a Nutritional Supplement on Liver Function Tests and Midluteal Serum Steroid Levels in Women with Premenstrual Tension Syndromes." *Journal of Applied Nutrition,* March 1985.

Goei, G. S.; Ralston J. L.,; and Abraham, Guy E. "Dietary Patterns of Patients with Premenstrual Tension." *Journal of Applied Nutrition,* Vol. 34, No. 1.

Hutchens, Alma R. *Indian Herbology of North America.* London: Garden City Press Ltd., 1973.

Mukerjee, Chunilal. "Premenstrual Tension: A Critical Study of the Syndrome." *Journal of the Indian Medical Assn.,* Vol. 24, No. 3.

Piesse, John W. "Nutrition Factors in the Premenstrual Syndrome." *International Clinical Nutrition Review,* Vol. 4, No. 2.

Timonen, Sakari, and Procope, Berndt-Johan. "Premenstrual Syndrome and Physical Exercise." *Acta. Obstet. Gynec. Scand,* Vol. 50: pp. 331–337.

THE STRENUOUS EXERCISER'S DIET

Bailey, Covert. *Fit or Fat.* Boston: Houghton Mifflin, 1978.

Bland, Jeffrey, ed. *Medical Applications of Clinical Nutrition.* New Canaan, Conn.: Keats Publishing, 1983.

Christensen, Kim. *Sports Nutrition.* Houston: International Preventative Medicine Foundation, 1984.

Coleman, Ellen. *Eating for Endurance.* California Dietetic Association, P.O. Box 3506, Santa Monica, Calif. 90403.

Glover, Bob, and Shepherd, Jack. *The Runner's Handbook.* New York: The Viking Press, 1978.

Goodhart, Robert S., and Shils, Maurice E. *Modern Nutrition in Health and Disease,* 6th ed. Philadelphia: Lea & Febiger, 1980.

Hecker, Arthur L., ed. *Clinics in Sports Medicine: Symposium on Nutritional Aspects of Exercise.* Philadelphia: W. B. Saunders, Vol. 3, No. 3.

Higdon, Hal, ed. *The Complete Diet Guide for Runners and Other Athletes.* Mountain View, Calif.: World Publications, 1978.

Lamb, David R. "Anabolic Steroids in Athletics: How Well Do They Work and How Dangerous Are They?" *The American Journal of Sports Medicine,* Vol. 12, No. 1.

Pipes, Dr. Thomas. "Over-the-Counter Drugs." *Runner's World,* December 1979.

Strauss, Richard H., ed. *Sports Medicine.* Philadelphia: W. B. Saunders Co., 1984.

Zeno, Ken. "Sports and Nutrition: The Invisible Connection." *Whole Life Times,* July/Aug., 1982.

Zuckerman, Sam. "Food for Sport." *Nutrition Action,* July/Aug., 1984.

THE BIRTH CONTROL PILL DIET

Buist, Robert A. "Drug-Nutrient Interactions—An Overview." *International Clinical Nutrition Review,* Vol. 4, No. 3.

Herxheimer, Andrew. "Immortality for Old Drugs?" *The Lancet,* Vol. 1, No. 8392.

Roe, Daphne. *Drug-Nutrient Interactions.* Hoffman-La Roche, Inc., product information sheet number c.

Weiss, Kay, ed. *Women's Health Care: A Guide to Alternatives.* Reston, Va.: Prentice-Hall, 1984.

THE CAFFEINE-USER'S DIET

Please see the references in The Cyst and Tumor Diet and the Pregnancy Diet.

THE SOCIAL DRINKER'S DIET

Halsted, Charles H. "Nutritional Implications of Alcohol." *Nutrition Reviews' Present Knowledge in Nutrition,* 4th ed. Washington, D.C.: The Nutrition Foundation, 1976.

Ketcham, Katherine, and Mueller, L. Ann. *Eating Right to Live Sober.* Seattle: Madrona Publishers, 1983.

Korsten, Mark A., and Lieber, Charles S. "Nutrition and the Alcoholic." *Medical Clinics of North America,* Vol. 63, No. 5.

Poulos, C. Jean; Stoddard, Donald; and Carron, Kathryn. *The Relationship of Stress to Hypoglycemia and Alcoholism.* Huntington Beach, Calif.: International Institute of Natural Health Sciences, 1976.

Roe, Daphne A. *Drug-Induced Nutritional Deficiencies.* Westport, Conn.: AVI Publishing Co., 1980.

Williams, Roger J. *Nutrition Against Disease.* Huntington Beach, Calif.: International Institute of Natural Health Sciences.

THE SMOKER'S DIET

"Dietary Beta-Carotene—An Anti-Cancer Agent?" *International Clinical Nutrition Review,* July, 1983.

Ketcham, Katherine, and Mueller, L. Ann. *Eating Right to Live Sober.* Seattle: Madrona Publishers, 1983.

"Medical Digest." *Health and Longevity Report,* Vol. 2, No. 10.

"Smokers Have an Increased Need for Vitamin C." *The Nutrition Report,* Vol. 2, No. 9.

THE STRESSFUL LIVING DIET

Kaplan, Jane Rachel. *A Woman's Conflict: The Special Relationship Between Women and Food.* New Jersey: Prentice-Hall, 1980.

Pelletier, Kenneth R. *Healthy People in Unhealthy Places: Stress and Fitness at Work.* New York: Delacorte Press, 1984.

INDEX

AA. *See* Alcoholics Anonymous
Abraham, G., 2, 3, 7, 9, 38, 41, 74, 107, 113, 140, 145
  article on calcium by, 140
Acidophilus, 127, 128
Acne, 112
  supplements for, 114
Acupuncture, 7, 78, 84. *See also* "Auxiliary treatment" under specific condition
  liver and, 35
Additives and preservatives, 67–68
Additives chart, 68
Adolescence and hormonal changes, 6–7
Adrenalin, 65
Adrenals, 66, 81, 86, 89, 95
  dizziness and, 36
  eyes and, 36
  knee problems and, 37
Aerobic exercise, 33, 80
Alcohol, 31, 66–67, 80–81, 83, 157
  auxiliary treatment for, 84
  diet to counteract, 80–84
  health problems caused by, 66, 140
  supplements to take for, 83–84
  vitamins lost when drinking, 66
Alcoholics Anonymous (AA), 82, 84, 104
Alcoholism, 81
  diet to counteract, 80–84
  nutritional deficiencies caused by, 82
Aldosterone, 37, 147
  allergies and, 37, 86, 104, 109
  cortisol and, 37
Alslaben, H., 66
Aluminum
  cooking utensils, 54
  diseases associated with, 52, 54
Alzheimer's disease, 52
Amenorrhea, 41
  auxiliary treatment for, 123
  causes of, 43
  diet for, 120
  supplements for, 122–123
  types of, 120

American Meat Institute, 5
Amines, 104, 105, 106
Amino acids, 77, 151, 152
  arginine, 152
  l-arginine and herpes, 133
  l-glutamine, 81–82, 83, 149
  l-lysine, 132, 133, 134
  ornithine, 152
  osteoporosis and, 152
  precautions when taking, 77
  supplements, 77
  tyrosine, 149, 150
Anemia, 49, 101, 154
Anorexia, 115–117
  diet for, 115–117
  supplements for, 117
  support groups for, 119
Antacids, 3, 101, 103
Antibiotics, 29, 30, 42
  infections and, 30
Antifungal agents, 125, 127, 128
Antifungal tea, 128
Anti-illness diet, 44–70, 71
  problems addressed by, 10, 37
  recipes for, 57–62
Anxiety, 145
Arthritis, 3, 37, 91, 139, 140
  aspirin and, 92
  auxiliary treatment for, 94
  dairy products and, 90, 92
  diet for, 90–94
  eggs and, 91
  foods to avoid and, 90–91
  nightshade family and, 90, 91, 92
  pain relief for, 92, 94
  supplements for, 93–94
  types of, 90
  vitamins for, 91
Ascorbic acid. *See* Vitamin C
Aspartame, 97
Aspirin, 92, 110
Atherosclerosis, 3, 139
  blood sugar and, 95
Auxiliary treatment, general types of, 77–80

Back pain, 37
Barbash, H., 137
Barley, 46
Basic Four food groups, 4, 5
Beans, 47, 134
Benson, H., 134

Beta carotene, 127, 128, 158, 159
Betaine hydrochloride, 76, 103
Beverages and meals, 54
Biermann, J., 97, 99
Biochemical individuality, 20, 24–43
Biofeedback, 79, 108, 139
Bioflavinoids, 73, 74
Biotin, 74, 111, 112, 114, 154, 155
Birth control pill(s), 41, 42, 143
  anemia and, 154
  diet to counteract effects of, 1, 154–155
  supplements for, 155
  vitamins and, 7
Bland, J., 9, 50, 73, 131, 142
Blood pressure, 66, 67
  foods that lower, 107
Blood serum, 92, 103
Blood sugar, 36, 63, 65, 66, 81, 99
  diet for problems related to, 94–99
  eating to prevent low, 36
  food cravings and, 81
  foods that affect, 94
  fructose and, 97
  legumes and, 47, 98
  marijuana and, 95
  pasta and, 96
  sugars and, 71, 97
  supplements for, 99
  symptoms of imbalance of, 17, 36
Bone, 65. *See also* Osteoporosis
  loss of, 3, 7, 141
Brain scan, 107
Bran, 46
Breakfast, 51–52,
  recipes for, 54–55
Breasts
  cancer of the, 129, 130
  cysts in, 129, 130
  insulin and tissue of the, 130, 131
Brewer's yeast, 84, 99, 149, 151, 155, 157, 158
Bromelain-papain, 76
Buckwheat, 46
Bulimia, 38
  auxiliary treatment for, 119
  diet for, 117

support groups for, 119–120

Butter (better) recipe, 57

Caffeine, 4, 26, 106, 140, 141
  breast cysts and, 130, 156
  diet to counteract effects of, 155–157
  effects of, 31, 64–65
  supplements for users of, 156–157
Calcification, 90, 91
  solanin and, 90
Calcium, 3, 4, 7, 9, 38, 45, 50, 52, 54, 65, 66, 75, 91, 100, 101, 117, 139, 140–141, 143, 146, 155, 157, 158
  controversy about, 1, 2
  malabsorption of, 2, 3, 92, 139, 140–141
  osteoporosis and, 140
  soft drinks and, 65–66
Calcium deposits, 38
Calories, 8
Candida albicans, 30, 38, 124
  antibiotics and, 30
  auxiliary treatment for, 129
  causes of, 42
  diet for, 124–129
  foods to avoid for, 125, 128
  homeopathic remedy for, 125
  supplements for, 127–128
  symptoms of, 39–40, 124–125
  treatment for, 125
Carbohydrates, 5, 8, 70, 71, 95, 98, 101, 102, 131, 157
Carob, 131
Center for Science in the Public Interest, 68
Cheraskin, E., 9, 63
Chicken recipe, 61
Childers, N., 90
Chiropractors, 78. See also "Auxiliary treatment" under specific condition
Chocolate, 141
Cholesterol, 63, 110
  acceptable levels of, 110
Choline, 99
Chromium, 75, 96, 97
Cleft palate, 143
Clinical ecology, 90
Clorox, 106
Coca, A., 87
Cocaine, 30
Coffee substitutes, 54

Cola drinks, 65
Cold-pressed vegetable oils, 51
Cold sores, 40, 42
Colitis, 35
Collagen, 92, 94
Colon, 35
  caffeine and, 65
  iceberg lettuce and, 48
Compulsive eating, 117–120
Contraceptives. See Birth control pill(s); Intrauterine device
Cooking utensils
  avoid aluminum, 52, 54
  preferred, 54
Copper, 7, 49, 74, 92, 94, 112, 114
Corn, 46
Cortisol, 37
Council for Responsible Nutrition (CRN), 73
Cramps. See Menstrual cramps
Craving for foods, 20
Creighton, J., 79
Crook, W., 85
Cysts and tumors, 129–132
  auxiliary treatment for, 132
  diet for, 129–132
  drugs to avoid for, 130
  foods to avoid for, 130, 131
  vitamin E and, 110, 130, 131

Dairy products, 4, 32, 49, 145
  diet free of, 88
Decaffeinated coffee, 65
Depression, 36, 149
Dermatitis, 112, 114
DES (diethylstilbestrol), 26
Diabetes, 65, 94, 95
  diet for, 98–99
  fructose and, 97
  high fiber diet and, 98, 99
  pasta and, 98
  sugars and, 97
  symptoms of, 97
  types of, 96
Diamond, S., 105
Digestion, 37, 100
  auxiliary treatment for, 103
  diet for good, 100–103
  HCL deficiency and, 34
  poor, 1, 2, 32, 35, 85–86, 112
  water-soluble vitamins and, 113
  stools as indicators of poor, 34, 35
  supplements for good, 94, 103

Digestive aids, 75, 76, 94
Dinner, 53
  recipes for, 55–56
Diseases linked to specific foods, 4
Diuretics, 117, 147
Diverticulitis, 35
Dizziness, 36
Dong, C., 90
Dopamine, 145
Drinker's (social) diet, 157–158
Drinking liquids with meals, 32, 54
Drugs, chemicals, and health, 30
Dry form of vitamins recommended over oil-based form, 130, 131, 158
Dry skin, 112–113, 114

Eating disorders, 38
  auxiliary treatment for, 120
  diet for, 115–120
  support groups for, 119–120
Eating habits, 103
  ways to change, 23
Eating out, 55–56, 69–70
Edelstein, C., 120
Ellis, J., 143
Endocrine glands, 151
Enzymes, 34, 83, 89, 90, 93, 100, 101, 103, 105, 112, 127
Enzyme therapy, 89
Essential fatty acids (EFAs), 2, 50, 51, 62, 73, 100, 111–113, 115–116, 148
  deficiency of, 51
Estrogen, 113, 120, 121, 145
Estrogen therapy, 7
Exercise, 80, 141, 176
Exerciser's diet, 14, 150–154
Eyes, 36
  liver and, 35

Family, health problems running in, 24, 96, 106
Fatigue, 32, 103–104
  diet for, 103–104
Fats, 49, 50–51, 62, 110
  types of, 62
  cheese low in, 49
Fats and oils, 50–51, 62–63, 69
  types of, 62
FDA. See Food and Drug Administration

Fiber
  diabetes and, 98–99
  diet high in, 98, 99
  varicose veins and, 35
Folic acid, 7, 49, 66, 75, 81,
    84, 89, 109, 143, 144,
    154, 155, 157
Food addictions, 85
Food allergies, 85–86
  auxiliary treatment for, 90
  diet for, 85–90, 118
  foods to avoid in, 85
  supplements for, 89–90
  symptoms of, 21–22
  vitamins for, 89
Food and Drug Administration
    (FDA), 5, 73
Food combining, 5, 101, 102
Food cravings, 20, 81, 85,
    117, 148
Food intolerance, 18, 19, 20–
    22
Food reactions. *See* Food in-
    tolerance
Foods
  avoid these, 62–69
  "cool," types of, 122
  disease-promoting, 4
  preferred, 68–69
  rotation of, 87
  slower digesting, 18
  "warm," types of, 122
  varying, 87
Food substitution, 68
Ford, N., 134
Fredericks, C., 92
Fructose, 50, 97, 98, 99
Fruit, 5, 6, 50
  best way to eat, 50
  cysts or tumors and, 131
  juices from, 50
  when to avoid, 5, 50

Gall bladder, 35, 141
Gallstones, 141
Genetic predisposition to
    health problems, 24
Glandular supplements, 108,
    111, 134, 157, 160
Glandular therapy, 76–77
Glucose, 97, 151
Glucose tolerance test, 96
Glycemic index, 96, 97, 98
Goodhart, R., 140, 151
Gout and vitamin C, 110
Grains, 44–47, 49
Guarana herb, 65

Headaches, 106, 107
  auxiliary treatment for,
    107–108

caffeine and, 106
diet for, 104–108
foods that cause, 105–106
foods to avoid for, 105
migraine, 106–108
monosodium glutamate and,
    105
premenstrual, 107
situations that cause, 37
spinach and, 105
sulfur and, 107
supplements for, 107
Health diary, 11–23
Health, Education, and Wel-
    fare, Department of
    (HEW), 5
Health history
  family, 24–27
  personal, 27–38
  questionnaires, 25–38
Health practitioner, choosing
    a, 162–163
Health premises, primary, 2
Health problems helped by
    anti-illness diet, 10
Heart disease, 47, 151
Hemorrhoids, 35
Herb tea, 82, 160
Herbs, 8, 65
Herpes, 40, 42, 132–135
  auxiliary treatment for,
    134–135
  diet for, 132–135
  supplements for, 134
Heuser, G., 105
Heyden, S., 5
Higdon, H., 153
High fat diet, 4, 141
High fiber diet, 98, 99
Hills, H., 88
Hirsch, S., 88
Homeopathic preparation,
    129
Honey, 63
Hormones, 41
  adrenalin, 36
  aldosterone, 37
  cortisone, 36
Horrobin, D., 115, 130
Human Nutrition Institute, 63
Hummus recipe, 59–60
Hydrochloric acid (HCL), 2,
    3, 66, 78, 81, 86, 89,
    90, 92, 100, 101, 103,
    117, 122, 123, 140,
    141
  inhibitors of, 100–101
  symptoms of lack of, 34
Hyperglycemia, 80
Hypoglycemia, 65, 80, 94, 96,
    98

auxiliary treatment for, 99
controversy over diet for,
    49, 97
diet for, 98–99
symptoms of, 96
types of, 95–96

Iceberg lettuce, 48, 159
Immune system, 37, 42, 110
  auxiliary treatments for,
    111
  cell types of, 108
  depressors of, 109
  diet for, 108–111
  supplements for, 111
  vitamins for, 93–94
Inositol, 99
Insecticides, removal of, 106
Insulin, 95, 99
  breast tissue and, 130, 131
Intestines, 35
Iodine, 7, 75
Iron, 47, 65, 75, 81, 91, 92,
    94, 100, 101, 104, 110,
    143, 144, 151
IUD (intrauterine device),
    138, 151

Jenkins, D., 96
Jones, M., 88
Juices, fruit, 50

Kalita, D., 87, 89
Kasha, 46
Kaufman, W., 91
Ketcham, K., 83
Ketoacids, 148
Kidneys, 141, 148
Kidney stones, 141
  vitamin C and, 110
Kinesiology, 78
Kirschman, J., 112
Knee problems and adrenals,
    37

Lactose, 145
Laiken, D., 137
Lappé, F., 48, 102
Laxatives, 117
Lead toxicity, 150
Legumes, 44, 47, 49, 98
  hypoglycemia and, 98
Lentils, 47
Lettuce, types of, 48
Levin, A., 85
Light-headedness, 49
Linus Pauling Institute, 9, 73
Linus Pauling Seal of Quality,
    9, 73
Liquids and meals, 32

Liver, 82, 95, 151, 157
  causes of damage to, 35
  functions of, 35
  organic, 151, 157, 158
London, R., 130
Low blood pressure and sulfur, 107
Low fat diet, 98
Lunch, 52–53
  recipes, 55
Lymph nodes, 108

MacHovec, F., 79
Magee, K., 107
Magnesium, 2, 3, 4, 7, 9, 45, 50, 52, 74, 75, 91, 94, 138, 140, 141, 145, 146, 147, 148, 149, 150, 157
Mandell, F., 87, 88
Mandell, M., 87
Margarine, 51, 62
Marijuana and blood sugar, 30, 95
Marshall, J., 80, 137
Massage. See "Auxiliary treatment" under specific condition
May, C., 85
McGovern, G., Senator, 5
Meat, 34, 67
Medications, 25
Megavitamin therapy, 82
Menopause, 7, 8, 40, 42
  auxiliary treatment for, 137
  diet for, 135–137
  supplements for, 136
  symptoms of, 7, 37, 40–41, 135–136
Menstrual cramps, 137
  auxiliary treatment for, 139
  diet for, 137
  evening primrose oil and, 138
  supplements for, 138
Menstrual cycle and PMS, 12
Menstruation, 7, 135
Migraines, 106–107
  acupuncture and, 107
  causes of, 107
Millet, 47, 57
Minerals. See specific mineral
Mineral water, 66, 159
Miso, 122
Monilia, 30
Mononucleosis, 26
Monosodium glutamate (MSG), 67, 104, 105
  foods that contain, 67
Morning sickness, 142
Morton, R., 115

MSG. See Monosodium glutamate
Mueller, L., 83

Napoli, M., 130
National Migraine Foundation, 105
National Nutritional Foods Association (NNFA), 73
Niacin, 14, 94, 107, 111, 112
Niacinamide, 74, 75, 91, 92, 138, 148
Nitrites, 67
Nitrosamines, 67
Nittler, A., 77
Nonken, P., 88
Nutrition, new (the), 1
Nuts, 49, 50
  difficult to digest, 50
  rancidity and, 50
Nuts and seeds, 50
  types of, 50

Oatmeal, 52, 58
Oats, 46
Obesity, 99
Oils, 2, 51, 62, 114, 127, 128, 138, 148, 149
  rancidity of, 73
  recommended, 68, 69
  types of vegetable, 62–63
On Course, Inc., 79
Optivite, 74–77, 114, 141
  where to purchase, 74
  vitamin and mineral dosages in, 74–77
Orthomolecular medicine, 6, 35, 43, 122
Osteopath, 90, 105, 107
Osteoporosis, 3, 7, 40, 42, 43, 54, 65, 101, 139–142, 152
  auxiliary treatment for, 142
  causes of, 139, 140
  diet for, 139–142
  exercise and, 141
  foods to avoid with, 140
  supplements for, 141–142
Oxylalic acid, 140, 141, 142

Pancake recipe, 57
Pancreas, 34, 95, 96, 100, 101, 112
  enzymes of, 83, 89, 90, 100, 101, 103, 112, 127
Parkinson's disease, 54
Pasta recipe, 60, 96, 98
Pauling, Linus (Institute), 9
Peanuts, 47
Peas, 47, 134
Pelletier, K., 160

Pelvic inflammatory disease (PID), 138
Pesticides, removal from food, 106
Pfeiffer, C., 9, 91, 107
Philpott, W., 9, 87, 89
Phosphorus, 3, 66, 140, soft drinks and, 65–66
Phytates, 49
Pituitary gland, 36, 135
PMS. See Premenstrual syndrome
PMT. See Premenstrual tension
Politics and nutrition, 4–5
Popcorn recipe, 61–62
Potassium, 4, 37, 75, 117
Potatoes, 71, 92
Pots and pans, aluminum, 52, 54
Porman, R., 87
Porrath, S., 130
Postpartum blues, 143
Pregnancy, 142
  auxiliary treatment for, 144
  diet for, 142–144
  supplements for, 144
  vitamins required during, 7, 142–143
Premenstrual syndrome, 3, 9, 12, 86, 107, 137, 144–150. See also Premenstrual tension
  auxiliary treatment for, 146, 148–149, 150
  causes of, 41–42, 145
  diet for, 144–150
  foods to avoid for, 145
  supplements for, 146
  support groups for, 147
  symptoms of, 7, 37–39, 145–146
  types of, 41–42, 145–147
Premenstrual tension, 144–150. See also Premenstrual syndrome
  supplements for, 146, 148, 149, 150
  symptoms of, 39
  types of, 39, 147–150
Preservatives and additives, 67
Primrose oil, 139, 149
Pritikin Diet, 51
Progesterone, 113, 120, 143, 145, 150
Progesterone therapy, 41
Prostaglandins, 51, 148
  cramps and, 137
Protein, 6, 7, 101, 102, 153
  complete, 49

digestion time for, 53
eating too much, 48–49
Protein combining, 49
Protein drinks, 52
recipe for, 58–59
Proteolytic enzymes, 89
Psychotherapy, 78–79. *See also* "Auxiliary treatment" under specific condition
Ptyalin, 100, 103
Puhl, J., 151
Pulse test, 86–87
Pyridoxine, 7, 74, 75, 84, 89, 91, 92, 94, 109, 111, 138, 141, 142, 143, 144, 145, 146, 147, 148, 150, 154, 155

Rancidity and EFAs, 113
RDA. *See* Recommended Daily Allowance
Recipes, 57–62
breakfast, 54–55
dinner, 55–56
lunch, 55
Recommended Daily Allowance (RDA), 8, 158
Recommended dosages of vitamins and minerals, 74–77
Recovering alcoholic, diet for, 80–84
Reiser, S., 63
Relaxation tapes, 79
Reproductive system, 29, 42
diets for, 120, 154
Riboflavin, 74, 75, 84
Rice, 45–46
Rotation diet, 87
Russo, G., 90
Rye, 46

Salicylate, 110
Salt, 32, 37
Saper, J., 107
Sauna, 114
Scanlon, W., 87
Seely, S., 63, 130
Selenium, 75, 81, 110, 127
Senate report on diet, 4–5
Sensitivities to food. *See* Food intolerance
Serotonin, 118
Sesame seeds, 50
Shils, M., 140, 151
Shute, W., 66
Simonton, C., 79
Simonton, S., 79
Skin, 1, 36, 113
auxiliary treatment for, 114

diet for, 111–114
supplements for, 114
Skin, poultry, 68
Smog and beta carotene, 158
Smokers, diet for, 158–159
supplements for, 159
Smoking, 31, 140, 158
Snacks, 53, 56
Soba noodles, 61
Social drinker's diet, 157–158
supplements for, 158
Society for Clinical Ecology, 90
Sodium, 4, 37, 66, 148
soft drinks and, 65–66
mineral water low in, 66
Sodium nitrates and nitrites, 67
Soft drinks, 65–66
Solanin, 90
Soya, 49, 52, 67
milk recipe from, 57–58
Spine, 29, 90, 144
Spleen, 108
Sports, 8
Steam room, 114
Steroids, 152
Stools, 34, 35
Strenuous exerciser's diet, 150–154
supplements for, 153
Stress, 36, 37, 65, 66, 81, 104, 109, 145
auxiliary treatment for, 160
diet for, 159–161
supplements for, 160
vitamins needed for, 8
Sucrose, 63
Sugar, 32, 63–64, 140
craving for, 81
fruit and, 5
types of, 63
water retention and, 147
Sulfur, 91, 107
foods that contain, 107
headaches and, 107
Supplements, 72, 73–77. *See also* "Supplements" under specific condition
Surgery, 29
Sweeteners, preferred, 68
Synovial fluid, 90

Tabbouli, 60, 96
Taheebo tea, 128
Tapes, relaxation, 79
Teflon, 52
Thiamine, 74, 75, 81, 84, 157
Thymus gland, 108, 111
Tofu, 47, 49, 59, 155
Toohey, B., 97, 99

Triglycerides, 63, 66
Triticale, 47
Truss, O., 106, 124–125
Tubal ligation, 41
Tumors, 130–131
auxiliary treatment for, 132
diet for tumors and cysts, 129–132
Tyson & Associates, 73, 77

USDA (United States Department of Agriculture), 4, 5, 63, 73

Vaginitis, 124
Varicose veins, 35
Vegetable oils, 51, 148
Vegetables, benefits of, 47–48, 61
Vegetable slaw recipe, 57
Vegetarianism, 49
Vinegar, 125
Vitamins, 66, 74–77. *See also* Vitamins, specific
dry form of, 72, 73, 158
malabsorption of, 112–113
recommended form of, 72, 73
recommended ratios and potencies, 74–75
Vitamins, specific
A, 66, 74, 84, 110, 111, 112, 114, 158, 159
toxicity and, 110
B complex, 7, 8, 50, 75, 80, 81, 84, 89, 94, 103, 112, 123, 125, 134, 149, 150, 151, 156, 158, 159, 160
alcohol and, 80, 125
recommended dosages of, 75
B_1. *See* Thiamine
B_2. *See* Riboflavin
B_3. *See* Niacin
B_6. *See* Pyridoxine
B_{12}, 7, 49, 74, 75, 81, 89, 109, 122, 154, 155, 157
C, 8, 67, 72, 73, 74, 84, 89, 91, 92, 94, 99, 109, 110, 111, 127, 128, 134, 135, 136, 138, 148, 151, 155, 158, 159, 160
toxic levels of, 67, 110
D, 7, 74, 90, 91, 93, 140, 142
E, 7, 73, 91, 93, 94, 110, 111, 113, 114, 127,

128, 130, 131, 135, 136, 151, 153, 155
breast cysts and, 110, 131
dry form of, 73, 130, 131
rancidity and, 113
synthetic, dry, 131
toxic levels of, 110
Vomiting, 117

Walford, R., 110
Water, 36, 113, 151
daily requirement of, 32
meals and water, 32, 54
retention of, 147

therapy, 135
vitamins soluble in, 113
Wheat, 18, 45
Wheat-free diet, 89
Wheat germ and rancidity, 45, 73
White flour and rice, 64
White sugar. See Sugar
Whole grains, 142
Williams, R., 8, 9, 20, 50, 81, 83
Wine, 157, 159, 160, 166
meals and, 103
Wrinkles, 113
supplements for, 114

Wurtman, J., 118

Yeast-free diet, 89
Yeast infection, 38
Yoga, 79–80, 161

Zellerbach, M., 85
Zinc, 7, 49, 66, 74, 80, 81, 91, 93, 94, 96, 99, 110, 111, 112, 114, 115–116, 143, 148, 155
deficiencies of, 49
RNA (ribonucleic acid) and, 112
sources of, 115

3, 5, 20,